THE CHALLENGE OF SEXUALITY IN
HEALTH CARE

THE CHALLENGE OF SEXUALITY IN HEALTH CARE

Hazel Heath and Isabel White

b

Blackwell Science

© 2002 by
Blackwell Science Ltd
Editorial Offices:
Osney Mead, Oxford OX2 0EL
25 John Street, London WC1N 2BS
23 Ainslie Place, Edinburgh EH3 6AJ
350 Main Street, Malden
   MA 02148 5018, USA
54 University Street, Carlton
   Victoria 3053, Australia
10, rue Casimir Delavigne
   75006 Paris, France

Other Editorial Offices:

Blackwell Wissenschafts-Verlag GmbH
Kurfürstendamm 57
10707 Berlin, Germany

Blackwell Science KK
MG Kodenmacho Building
7–10 Kodenmacho Nihombashi
Chuo-ku, Tokyo 104, Japan

Iowa State University Press
A Blackwell Science Company
2121 S. State Avenue
Ames, Iowa 50014-8300, USA

The right of the Author to be identified as the
Author of this Work has been asserted in
accordance with the Copyright, Designs and
Patents Act 1988.

First published 2002

Set in 10.5/12.5pt Palatino
by DP Photosetting, Aylesbury, Bucks
Printed and bound in Great Britain by
MPG Books Ltd, Bodmin, Cornwall

The Blackwell Science logo is a trade mark of
Blackwell Science Ltd, registered at the United
Kingdom Trade Marks Registry

DISTRIBUTORS

Marston Book Services Ltd
PO Box 269
Abingdon
Oxon OX14 4YN
(*Orders:*   Tel: 01235 465500
             Fax: 01235 465555)

USA
Blackwell Science, Inc.
Commerce Place
350 Main Street
Malden, MA 02148 5018
(*Orders:*   Tel: 800 759 6102
             781 388 8250
             Fax: 781 388 8255)

Canada
Login Brothers Book Company
324 Saulteaux Crescent
Winnipeg, Manitoba R3J 3T2
(*Orders:*   Tel: 204 837-2987
             Fax: 204 837-3116)

Australia
Blackwell Science Pty Ltd
54 University Street
Carlton, Victoria 3053
(*Orders:*   Tel: 03 9347 0300
             Fax: 03 9347 5001)

A catalogue record for this title is available from
the British Library

ISBN 0-632-04804-2

Library of Congress
Cataloging-in-Publication Data
The Challenge of sexuality in health care/[edited
by] Hazel Heath and Isabel White.
      p. ; cm.
      Includes bibliographical references and
index.
      ISBN 0-632-04804-2
      1. Holistic nursing – Great Britain.   2. Sex
(Psychology)   3. Nurse and patient.   I. Heath,
Hazel B.M.   II. White, Isabel.
      [DNLM: 1. Holistic Nursing.   2. Sexuality,
3. Nurse–Patient Relations.   4. Sex Behavior–
psychology. WY 86.5 C437 2001]
RT42.C435 2001
610.73–dc21   2001037815

For further information on
Blackwell Science, visit our website:
www.blackwell-science.com

Contents

Contents

Contributors

Hazel Heath, MSc Advanced Clinical Practice (Older People), BA(Hons), DipNursing(London), Cert Ed, FETC, ITEC, RGN, RCNT, RNT is an Independent Consultant on nursing and older people. Hazel has written widely and given many conference presentations on sexuality in later life. Her MSc research explored how nurses work with older people's sexuality and her doctoral thesis highlights bodywork and sexuality as challenging aspects of the work of nurses and care assistants with older people in care homes. Hazel is a seasoned campaigner for the rights of older people and her current consultancy work incorporates a range of national level projects. She is the editor of *Nursing Older People* journal and this is her fourth book.

Isabel White, MSc Nursing, BEd(Hons) Nursing Education, Diploma Life Sciences Nursing, RGN, RSCN, RNT was Head of Undergraduate Studies at the Centre for Cancer and Palliative Care Studies, Institute of Cancer Research, London, and is currently Lecturer–Practitioner in cancer care, Institute of Health Sciences, City University and Barts and the London NHS Trust. Isabel's MSc research investigated nurses' construction of sexuality within a cancer care context. Her interest is primarily focused on the impact of cancer and cancer therapies on the sexual/intimate relationships of those living with cancer and other chronic and life-threatening conditions. She is currently studying a postgraduate diploma in psychosexual therapy with a view to conducting PhD research in this aspect of cancer care. Isabel is also currently a nurse member of the National Cancer Task Force.

Elizabeth Grigg, MA, BA, PGDip (edu), Dip PR, SRN, RNT, FPA Cert, is Principal Lecturer at the Institute of Health Studies, University of Plymouth (Somerset Centre). Elizabeth has qualifications in health and social care and has worked within the arena of sexual health, sexuality and sexual ill health in both Australia and the UK for many years. She set up the first family planning clinic in Rockhampton, Queensland and developed the first sexual education and sexual health promotion programmes within the many and diverse sectors of the Central Queensland community – an area the size of Britain. Some of her research was used successfully in promoting sexuality education within the whole state school system in Australia.

Amanda Keighley, MA, DipNursing, Adv Dip Counselling, CertEd, RNMH, RNT is Senior Lecturer in Public Health and Primary Care at St Martin's College, Lancaster. She has worked with people with learning disability in a wide variety of settings. Throughout her career Amanda has focused on enabling children and adults with learning disabilities and their carers to develop in how they relate to others, both in a personal and sexual context. She maintains her clinical practice as a learning disability nurse and a counsellor and currently runs a counselling service for children and adults with learning disability. Amanda is also a member of the Department of Health (England) learning disability nursing practice advisory group and has recently been appointed to the executive for the Association for Pastoral and Spiritual Care Counselling.

Danny Kelly, MSc, BSc, DN Cert, Onc Cert, PGCE, RN is Senior Nurse (Research & Development) at UCL Hospitals, London. Danny worked as a charge nurse in a sexual health clinic and then in acute cancer care before moving into nurse education. He is now involved in facilitating nursing research in an NHS Trust and is completing doctoral research exploring men's experiences of prostate cancer.

Brendan McCormack, DPhil(Oxon), BSc(Hons), PGCEA, RGN, RMN, Professor of Nursing Research, University of Ulster is Director of Nursing Research and Practice Development, Royal Hospitals Trust, Belfast. Brendan's current work focuses on the development of person-centred approaches to practice and he works with nurses in a variety of settings in developing this approach. He has a particular interest in maintenance of mind–body integrity and holistic practice, of which sexuality is an integral part.

Helen Roberts, MSc, PGDipEd, RGN is Lecturer in Nursing at the University of York. Helen has extensive experience in cancer nursing practice, management and education. She developed an interest related to facial disfigurement when working as a clinical nurse specialist with people with head and neck cancer and her continued interest is in nurses' attitudes and responses to differences and diversity in practice.

Liz Searle, MSc Nursing, RN, RNT is Head of Education at Macmillan Cancer Relief. Liz has worked in cancer and palliative care education and practice since 1990. She is currently employed by Macmillan to lead and develop their education strategy and manage the Macmillan National Institute of Education. She is also a non-executive director of her local primary care trust.

Philippa Sully, MSc, RN, RM, RHV, Cert Ed, RNT, FP Cert, CC Relate is Senior Lecturer in Interprofessional Practice at the Institute of Health Sciences, City University, London. Philippa's background is primary health care, women's health and counselling psychology. She worked for many years in the voluntary sector as a couples counsellor. As a practice-based academic Philippa is a consultant to a number of organisations and is course leader for the Interprofessional Practice MSc, 'Society, Violence and Practice'.

Barbara Walters, MSc, DipN(Lon), DipNE(Lon), RN, RM, RCNT, RNT is Reproductive and Sexual Health Pathway Leader at the Institute of Health Sciences, City University, London. Barbara has extensive experience in the practice and teaching of gynaecological nursing and is currently Chair of the Royal College of Nursing's Gynaecological Nursing Forum.

Martin F. Ward, MPhil, DipNursing, NEBSS Dip, Cert Ed, RMN, RNT is Independent Nurse Consultant and Director of MW Professional Development Limited. Martin has been a mental health nurse in different capacities from a practitioner, educator and researcher to the director of mental health for the Royal College of Nursing for over 30 years. During that time he has published extensively in the nursing press and spoken at conferences throughout the world. In all that time the subject of sexuality has remained as taboo for patient care as it has in society generally, yet it remains fundamental to the individual's self-identity. Martin's chapter has been written to raise practitioner awareness of the need to focus on the many aspects of patient sexuality in a mental health setting so that the 'missing link' of holistic care can be addressed with the sensitivity that it deserves.

Carole Webster, BSc(Hons), DipNursing, Dip Higher Ed (Biological Sciences), RGN, RM, RNT was Lecturer in Biological Sciences at St Bartholomew School of Nursing and Midwifery, London, where she taught on many aspects of sexuality particularly physiological and pharmacological. She is now a welfare rights adviser and has worked with a variety of charities. She advises on issues of access for people with disability and has developed advice on sexual activity for people with chronic pain. She has extensive first-hand experience of chronic illness and pain and is a wheelchair user.

Part 1
Sexuality – Concept, Context and Influences

Introduction

Isabel White and Hazel Heath

Sexuality and health care

One might be forgiven for assuming that sex is almost a national obsession. Sexuality has become an increasingly prominent topic within both the general media and nursing literature in Britain, with an explosion of both anecdotal and empirical accounts since the middle of the 1980s. During the sexual revolution of the 1960s issues of sex and sexuality increasingly moved into mainstream social consciousness. The emergence of HIV and AIDS in the 1980s was probably the most significant social influence on sexuality in that politically it moved sex, sexual behaviour and sexual orientation out of the wings to centre stage. At the time there were calls for a return to Victorian family values and a number of other legacies from the period are still the subject of debate today. The homophobic undercurrents within mainstream society became legitimised through the repeated rejection of calls to reduce the legal age of consent for gay men to that of heterosexuals, and legislation such as section 28 of the Local Government Act (1988) banned local authorities from intentionally promoting homosexuality. More recently, the continuing rise in teenage pregnancy rates has fuelled concerns over the nature of sex education within the national curriculum and controversy still rages over the decision to make emergency contraception (the morning after pill) available to adolescent girls through pharmacy outlets.

Sex and sexuality appear to be at one and the same time private to individuals or couples and yet part of the public discourse interwoven within the systems of religion, medicine and law that shape the fabric of modern society. Foucault was intrigued by this apparent paradox about sex in modern society:

'What is peculiar to modern societies, in fact, is not that they consign ... sex to a shadowy existence, but that they dedicate ...

3

themselves to speaking of it ad infinitum, while exploiting it as the secret.'

(Foucault, 1979, p.35)

Nurses are members of such a society with all its apparent double standards, hypocrisy, norms and mores. It is within this social context that nursing endeavours to provide care and services related to sexuality.

As practitioners have been encouraged to develop closer relationships with patients in the provision of what may be termed holistic care, sexuality has become worthy of nursing attention and action as a fundamental aspect of human experience in both health and illness. Sexuality has been publicly acknowledged as a legitimate aspect of health care through national policy initiatives such as the inclusion of sexual health as a key target area within the *Health of the Nation* strategy document (Department of Health, 1992). The Department of Health (DOH) and the Royal College of Nursing (RCN) are expected to publish revised sexual health strategies in 2001, recognising the continued importance of sexuality as a key facet of not only the nation's health but also of healthcare provision. Nursing has responded with caution to this enhanced societal focus through the work of its professional organisations. For example, the development of sexual health education and training guidelines by the English National Board (ENB, 1994), the launch of the Royal College of Nursing Sexual Health Forum in 2000 and publication of the College's first professional guidance document addressing sexuality and sexual health in nursing practice in the UK (RCN, 2000).

The purpose of the book

While the body of nursing literature that acknowledges sexuality is growing, much of this continues to be written in the absence of its social context or of an underpinning theoretical perspective. In addition the largely reductionist view offered by the psychological and biomedical sciences denies the fact that sexuality is inherently complex and socially constructed and thus cannot be adequately understood outwith its historical and cultural contexts (Foucault, 1979; Bancroft, 1989).

This book places sexuality in both these contexts, confronting the difficult and challenging realities of this social world for both nursing and wider society. The reader is offered a detailed exploration of the diverse and multiple perspectives of sexuality in contemporary nursing and health care, including their relevance to areas of nursing not always associated with the subject, such as child health and palliative care. Through appreciation of this context nurses can gain a better understanding of why sexuality often remains such a sensitive and difficult aspect of care to implement in practice. A strong theoretical perspective enables the nurse to appreciate the inherent challenges in addressing sexuality and can help to explain the feelings of embarrassment and inadequacy that often arise in nurses and patients when trying to tackle those issues in practice.

The book recognises the importance of sexuality and sexual health not only as a central element of holistic care, but also in that well informed, skilled practitioners who can respond to the sexuality inherent in everyday practice will inevitably contribute to the effective management of a whole range of sensitive healthcare challenges.

This book is also offered in support of a professional response to sexuality that should be a proactive, planned and considered approach as opposed to the adoption of what Nichols (1993) refers to as the 'psychological casualty model'. Sexuality and psychosexual practice is pertinent to the social, interpersonal and psychological aspects of an individual's health and wellbeing. Yet current evidence suggests we have marginalised its position within holistic care in much the same way as Nichols observed happens to psychological care provision in physical illness. Nichols argues that in the absence of pre-existing or planned schemes of psychological care, health services (particularly hospitals) and individual practitioners fall back on this 'casualty' model. As he explains:

> 'The assumption in the casualty model is that people in hospital are basically fine unless they externalise distress or show disturbed behaviour, in which case they are singled out and regarded as psychological casualties. In such cases an outside expert in the form of a psychologist or psychiatrist [or psychosexual therapist?] is called in to deal with the problem, or drugs suppress [the distress]. In other words, before receiving psychological assistance, a person needs the "ticket" of significant psychological distress; there is no attempt to prevent this distress in the first place.'
>
> (Nichols, 1993, p.47)

In providing psychosexual care we are not proposing the nurse act as an expert nor as a psychosexual therapist, but what we do suggest is that timely intervention by a skilled practitioner can often prevent the need for further, usually more intensive or protracted, intervention.

This book is particularly for nurses working in settings where sexuality may not be the primary focus of service or care, such as mental health or surgical care. It also offers insights for settings where sexuality is the dominant feature of health care, as in genito-urinary medicine or reproductive health. It is anticipated that other healthcare professionals may also find this text useful in provoking them to consider their unique contribution to psychosexual care within the context of the interdisciplinary healthcare team.

A principal reason for the focus of this text relates to the fact that until relatively recently most types of sexual dysfunction were assumed to be psychogenic. It is now believed however that organic factors may be involved in as many as 50% of cases, hence the need for nurses from a range of specialities to be aware of the impact of illness or disability and its treatment on sexual expression.

This book offers unique and challenging perspectives on what sexuality may mean to people with a health problem. Nurses have the potential to support people who are trying to live fulfilled lives, particularly when illness, disability or changes in circumstances threaten fundamental aspects of their sexual identity or lifestyle. Sensitivity, sound knowledge, advanced interpersonal skills, open-mindedness and flexibility are required in order to work effectively.

A variety of key themes run through the book, linking and providing synthesis for the diverse perspectives on sexuality contained within this multi-author text. The principal themes are:

- the public and private aspects of sexuality
- the issue of control through the 'nursing gaze' – care environments, nurses watching patients, patients watching nurses
- power – how the use and abuse of power is manifest through sexual stereotyping, prejudice and harassment
- gender issues in professional and intimate relationships
- the impact of being deemed asexual – those who are stigmatised by virtue of older age, disability, disfigurement, life-threatening illness
- 'controlling' and 'controlling out' sexual behaviour – the effects of care environments, access versus exclusion.

The book attempts to illustrate the complex array of influences upon the integration of sexuality within practical nursing care. Such issues include the age and gender of the nurse or patient, the need

for intimate body contact within the provision of care, the cc
or marginalisation of sexuality within a particular speciality or care
context and the impact of organisational and managerial cultures.

Defining sexuality

The concepts of sexuality and sexual health have generated a great
deal of discussion over recent years and many professionals have
had difficulty in finding a definition that captures the essential
components of human sexuality in the context of health and illness.
In addition it is becoming increasingly difficult to define sexual
health today, in a society where cultural and social boundaries and
expectations change very rapidly (ENB, 1994).

The World Health Organization (WHO, 1975) defines sexual
health as

> 'the integration of somatic, emotional, intellectual and social
> aspects of sexual being, in ways that are positively enriching and
> that enhance personality, communication and love'.

While difficult to attain for some practitioners, this concept of sexual health is one to which they can aspire in their psychosexual
work with patients and couples. Throughout this book, sexuality,
sexual expression and sexual health are considered in their broadest
sense and not merely defined as the absence of sexual dysfunction.

This text focuses on sexuality and sexual health as:

- an essential integrated element of the whole person
- embracing personal choice and tolerance of difference
- a creative force in human experience
- a fundamental aspect of how individuals relate to one another
- expressed by human beings in health, illness and disability
- expressed throughout the lifespan
- encompassing self-concept, sexual identity and sexual orientation
- encompassing psychological, social, cultural, spiritual and biological elements
- expressed through personal thoughts, feelings, behaviours, presentation, sensuality, intimacy and roles in life
- expressed negatively through power dynamics as in rape, sexual
  abuse and sexual harassment.

Structure of the book

The book is structured in four complementary parts that take the
reader on a journey from societal contexts of sexuality to the

microcosm of the nurse–patient relationship. The chapters are written by nurses working in the specific domains of nursing about which they write and their perspectives highlight the issues they consider important to their fields of work.

Part 1: Sexuality – Concept, Context and Influences

This first section sets the context for the book. It explores the construction of sexuality during three historical periods notable for the ways in which they portrayed sexuality as a troubled yet irresistible force in society and particularly for the legacy that has survived until today in the hearts, minds and sexual lives of contemporary Britain. This section also considers the influence of such social conventions related to sexuality upon nurses and nursing practice.

Chapter 1: Before the Sexual Revolution
Chapter 2: The Sexual Revolution
Chapter 3: Post HIV/AIDS: Emergence of a New Morality

Chapters 1–3 trace the social development of concepts of sexuality, plot the major influences on their construction and identify the key elements that remain as influences in contemporary society. The chapters explore the major mechanisms by which sexuality and sexual behaviour are defined and thus controlled: socio-cultural, including religion, medicine and the law; biological; and psychological.

Chapter 4: Nursing as a Sexualised Occupation
Chapter 5: Nurses, the Body and Body Work

These two chapters explore some of the reasons why nurses tend to avoid sexuality. Chapter 4 considers the societal values that imbue nursing (and nurses) with a sexual dimension and how this influences the organisation, management and practice of nursing. The controversial issue of sexual stereotyping as a mechanism of social control, prejudice and sexual harassment is considered.

Chapter 5 highlights why body work is an issue in nursing practice, together with some of the key challenges for nurses. It discusses how body work can become sexualised. It explores a range of perspectives on how the body has been viewed in literature and, specifically, the kinds of changes that people with illness or disability can experience.

Part 2: Sexuality through the Lifespan

This section addresses the development of sexuality and changing sexual priorities/issues across the lifespan. The chapters aim to offer a balanced view that encompasses the diversity of the UK population, in terms of lifestyle, sexual orientation and culture.

Chapter 6, Sexuality, Childhood and Adolescence, addresses normal and abnormal sexual development and the emergence of sexual identity. The chapter discusses sexual health education for children, particularly within the context of relationship development and explores the impact of sexual exploitation. It also examines possible reasons for avoidance and mystique in considering the sexuality of children.

Chapter 7, Sexuality and People with a Learning Disability, explodes the mythology surrounding the sexuality of people with a learning disability and considers the role of social education in the development of sexuality through structured support. Sex education, including risk management, is addressed together with the therapeutic strategies that can be used to manage the potential for power abuse in carer–client relationships and in reducing the person's vulnerability to exploitation and abuse.

Chapter 8, Sexuality, Fertility and Reproductive Health, represents sexuality in mid-life, particularly the promotion of couple bonding and intimacy through procreation. Fertility and transition to parenthood as a consequence of expressing sexuality are discussed in both their public and private aspects, together with the impact of infertility on sense of self.

Chapter 9, Sexuality and Later Life, analyses the construction of sexuality in later life and the factors influencing this. It explores some positive aspects of relationships in later life, alongside problems that may arise. The chapter concludes with suggestions on how the concept of sexuality might be reframed in older age and examples of how older people, and nurses who work with them, can help to overcome problems towards a more fulfilling expression of sexuality throughout later life.

Chapter 10, Sexuality and People who are Dying, explores the importance of intimacy, passion and commitment for those with life-limiting conditions and considers the impact of loss on sexuality. The relationship between media images of sex and death and the impact of these on patients and practitioners are discussed. This chapter asks whether or not the two taboo subjects in nursing remain sex and death and whether 'talking sex with angels' remains an unsurmountable challenge.

Part 3: Sexuality in Health and Illness

Each chapter focuses on a specific client group or area of health care and this part offers a range of views with a richness of perspectives. The chapters discuss areas of health care where sexuality is not uncommonly ignored because it is not perceived to be an issue for service users, for example because they do not readily conform to societal stereotypes of being young and beautiful. The chapters particularly focus on the experiences of people who have an illness or condition that stigmatises them, or one where the impact of disease, treatment or disability on their sexuality may not be recognised. A critique of care settings is offered and the impact of prevailing healthcare culture upon an individual's expressed needs versus what is deemed acceptable is explored. The role of the nurse as an agent of control and oppression is considered as well as her/ his capacity to manage difference, acknowledge difficult feelings, and to contribute to enhancement of a patient's self-esteem and sexuality.

Chapter 11: Sexuality and People with Mental Health Needs
Chapter 12: Sexuality and People Affected by Sexually Transmitted Infections
Chapter 13: Sexuality and People with Acute Illness
Chapter 14: Sexuality and People with Disability or Chronic Illness
Chapter 15: Sexuality and People with Disfigurement

Part 4: Current Approaches and Future Developments

Chapter 16, Facilitating Sexual Expression: Challenges for Contemporary Practice, offers a detailed analysis of the role of the nurse in psychosexual care through use of the P-LI-SS-IT model as a framework (Annon, 1976). Each of the four levels of nursing intervention is considered in turn and the contributions of individual practitioners, systems of care, care contexts and specialist agencies or psychosexual therapy are explored. Factors that facilitate or act as barriers to the provision of psychosexual care are discussed and practical examples of how nurses might improve professional care related to sexuality are offered.

Chapter 17 contains an overview of education and practice development recommendations, drawing together key themes in the book and highlighting the processes of knowledge and skills enhancement pertinent to this challenging domain of care.

While it could be tempting to offer prescriptions for psychosexual practice or tips for communicating about sexuality, such an approach not only demeans the complexity of the subjects, but also the sensitivity and courage of practitioners who are prepared to endure the discomfort of 'not knowing' in their support of patients. This book offers challenging perspectives on sexuality in health and ill health and no apologies are made for raising more questions than answers provided.

We hope this book encourages practitioners to work in partnership with patients and couples in offering a professional nursing response to psychosexual needs in health care.

As Peters (1972), a leading educational philosopher, asserted

'...to be educated [about sexuality in health care] is not to have arrived, but to travel with a different view.'

References

Annon, J. (1976) The P-LI-SS-IT model: a proposed conceptual scheme for behavioural treatment of sexual problems. *Journal of Sex Education Therapy*, **2**, 1–15.

Bancroft, J. (1989) *Human Sexuality and its Problems* (second edition). Churchill Livingstone, Edinburgh.

Department of Health (1992) *Health of The Nation*. DoH, London.

Department of Health (2001) The National Strategy for Sexual Health and HIV: Better Prevention: Better Services: Better Sexual Health, DoH, London.

English National Board for Nursing, Midwifery and Health Visiting (1994) *Sexual Health Education and Training, Guidelines for Good Practice in the Teaching of Nurses, Midwives and Health Visitors*. ENB, London.

Foucault, M. (1979) *The History of Sexuality*, Volume 1: An Introduction. Penguin Books, Harmondsworth.

Nichols, K. (1993) *Psychological Care in Physical Illness* (second edition). Chapman & Hall, London.

Peters, R.S. (1972) Education and the educated man. In: R.F. Deardon, P.H. Hirst & R.F. Peters (eds) *A Critique of Current Educational Aims*. Routledge & Kegan Paul, London.

Royal College of Nursing (2000) *Sexuality and Sexual Health in Nursing Practice*. RCN, London.

WHO (1975) Education and Trends in Human Sexuality: the training of health professionals, WHO Teaching Report Series No. 572. World Health Organization, Geneva.

1. *Before the Sexual Revolution*

Hazel Heath and Elizabeth Grigg

Sexuality is complex and therefore the study of sexuality is complex. Its multiple elements change over the course of time, as do the meanings ascribed to them. A range of approaches to exploring sexuality have been adopted but no single theory can encompass all its aspects. Sexuality has been studied from the perspectives of history, biology, psychology, sociology and across species and across cultures (Nevid *et al.*, 1995).

The usual assumption, according to Weeks (1989) is that

> '...sex is a definable and universal experience, with minority or unorthodox forms filtering off into tributaries which may, or more usually may not, be navigated by the conscious explorer' (p.1).

Weeks suggests, however, that it is the centrality given to this concept of sexuality that constitutes a problem for historians, for it ignores the great variety of cultural patterns that history reveals and the very different meanings given to what we blithely label as sexual activity.

According to Gagnon and Simon (1973), sexuality is subject to 'socio-cultural moulding to a degree surpassed by few other forms of human behaviour' (p.26). They also suggest that nothing is intrinsically sexual but anything can be sexualised within the influences of social interaction, social environment, culture and learned behaviour. Van Ooijen and Charnock (1994) ask 'what is a history of sexuality a history of?' other than a history of a subject which is in constant flux (Padgug, 1979; Weeks, 1989).

Michel Foucault describes sexuality as a web of relationships with complex elements; how these elements came together in particular practices might be termed sexuality. 'Sexuality must not be thought of as a kind of natural given force which power tries to hold in check, or as an obscure domain which knowledge tries gradually to uncover' (Foucault, 1979, p.105). Sex is also, according to Foucault, a historical construct. The elements of sexuality, including such notions as social, cultural and political behaviours, change over time. Within these perspectives, major mechanisms influence how sexuality and sexual behaviour are defined at any given moment. These include religion, the law, medicine, scientific writing and scholarship, including the work of the sexologists. Among the most crucial forms of mediation are the categories, concepts and languages which organise sexual life; which tell us what is good or bad, evil or healthy, normal or abnormal, appropriate or inappropriate behaviour. These too have a complex history (Weeks, 1985, p.7). By noting the construction of these elements at a particular point in time, it is possible to plot how they have developed and how these developments have influenced current thinking and the ways in which we construct our personal concepts of sexuality.

This chapter discusses selected topics which illustrate how the major elements and mechanisms of sexuality evolved during the course of history up to the mid twentieth century and concludes with examples of how present-day understanding of sexuality and sexual behaviour have been influenced by history. The chapter aims to provide a historical context for the chapters which follow.

Sociological and cultural perspectives

The evolution of the elements of sexuality and mechanisms by which it operates can be studied through the changes in major social and cultural aspects of life. Weeks (1989, p.15) suggests that these are as follows.

- *Kinship and family systems:* patterns of kinship and the organisation of family life and inheritance, class differences, the shaping of gender divisions.
- *Economic and social situations:* organisation of the economy, social environments and transformations, social situations of men and women (both ideologically and materially), work, patterns of courtship and relationships.
- *Forms of social regulation:* mechanisms of social regulation which may be formal (regulation by the church and state of marriage, divorce, illegitimacy, incest, sexual unorthodoxy etc, the welfare state), or informal (peer group regulation of adolescent courtship and sexual activity).

13

- *Political movements:* the political context in which decisions are made (e.g. to legislate or not, prosecute or ignore), instigation of moral panic.
- *Cultures of resistance:* cultures or sub-cultures which protest against prevailing moral codes or new momenta (e.g. against birth control, abortion, homosexuality, sexual liberation). These, according to Weeks (1989), are as much a part of history as the broader organisation of sexual codes.

Prevailing societal and cultural values define what is generally regarded as normal or abnormal, acceptable or unacceptable at any one time and can thus act as mechanisms of social control. Throughout history, different societies have developed varying standards for defining sexual values but some common themes can be identified. These are:

- Sex for procreation within an enduring relationship is valued. The enduring relationship, usually in the form of marriage, is also valued for the security it provides for offspring, maintaining and increasing the population, ensuring continuity of customs and passing valued property on to future generations.
- Sex in other relationships, for example sex outside marriage, polygamy, promiscuous sex, homosexuality and professional sex work, has been condemned by some societies and tolerated or encouraged by others.
- Incest has generally been regarded as taboo.
- Means of sexual expression such as masturbation have been viewed differently in different societies.

Social concepts of what is desirable/undesirable or moral/immoral not only influence and mould behaviour but they can transform the personal meaning ascribed to sexual activity or behaviour, as the following example illustrates:

'A married lady who is a leader in social purity movements and an enthusiast for sexual chastity discovered through reading some pamphlets against solitary vice that she had herself been practising masturbation for years without knowing it. The profound anguish and hopeless despair of this woman in the face of what she believed to be the moral ruin of her life cannot well be described.'

(Ellis, 1936, p.464)

14

As Weeks (1989, p.21) highlights, social definitions can make sexual what has hitherto seemed acceptable: harmless pleasure can become the gateway to nameless hells when, for whatever reasons, it begins to carry a significant symbolic meaning.

Religious influences

Throughout history, sexual expression and behaviour have been strongly influenced by religious codes, and continue to be so today.

The ancient Hebrews viewed sex in marriage as a fulfilling experience to strengthen the family and 'to be fruitful and multiply'. Homosexuality was condemned, as was adultery, particularly for women. Men owned the property and passed this onto their sons. Women were the property of their husbands and were taught to be 'good wives' (Telushkin, 1991).

The Islamic tradition treasures marriage and sexual fulfilment in marriage. The family is the backbone of Islamic society and celibacy is frowned upon (Ahmed, 1991). Men may take up to four wives but women are permitted only one husband. Women in most traditional Islamic societies are expected to keep their heads and faces veiled in public and to avoid all contact with men other than their husbands.

The Hindu culture cultivated sexual pleasure as a spiritual ideal. The *Kama Sutra*, believed to have been written at about the time that Christianity was developing as an organised religion, illustrates that sex was a religious duty and that sexual fulfilment was regarded as one way to reach a higher level of existence (Nevid *et al.*, 1995). It has been argued, however, that Indian society grew more restrictive towards sexuality after about AD 1000 (Tannahill, 1980).

According to the Christian Bible's New Testament, Jesus taught that love is paramount in human relations but little is known about Jesus's views on sex. Against a backdrop of sexual decadence among the upper classes in Rome, early Christian teachings began to associate sexuality with sin (Branden, 1981). The Christian church viewed virginity and sexual abstinence as the zenith of moral behaviour but later focused on procreative sex. Non-procreative sexual activity was considered sinful: this included masturbation, homosexuality, oral-genital contact and anal intercourse which were condemned. Nevid *et al.* (1995) suggest that to early Christians sexual pleasure, even within marriage, was stained by the original sin of Adam and Eve. In some eras it was even suggested that sex should be performed with one's spouse in the dark, removing as few clothes as possible. The idea, in either thought or action, of sex for pleasure and recreation, was adulterous and punishable by a penance.

In England, the revolution of Oliver Cromwell in 1649 saw the establishment of Puritanism in government. Sexual expression of any kind other than for procreation within marriage was condemned. Later, in the eighteenth century inhibition was reinforced by the Methodist movement, led by John Wesley. As the nineteenth century dawned any form of sexual expression was under tight restraint.

Sexually transmitted infections

Diseases with sexual connotations have historically carried with them not only prejudices that are linked to the state of knowledge at any one time but also the influences from the mores of the society of the day on sexual indulgence. Attitudes towards sexually transmitted infections (STIs) have changed continually.

In the sixteenth and seventeenth centuries, under the influence of Puritanism and Cromwell's Commonwealth in Britain, venereal diseases (VD) as they were then known, were feared and sufferers were isolated and described as 'loathsome and filthy' (Morton, 1976, p.120).

In the eighteenth century, described as an 'age of enlightenment', venereal diseases were less feared. Gonorrhoea and syphilis were common but did not appear to be life threatening in their early stages and there was no knowledge of the connection syphilis had to paralysis, heart disease, blindness and insanity. Sexual freedom was tolerated, to the extent that Casanova stated: 'there is no need of harlots in this fortunate age, so many decent women are as obliging as one could wish' (Morton, 1976, p.120).

The pendulum swung again in the nineteenth century. Venereal disease became sinful and degrading and became a penalty for straying from the 'path of good behaviour' (Morton, 1976, p.120). Laws were developed to curb the spread of diseases and isolate victims. For example, in 1864, the British government passed the Contagious Diseases Act which attempted to protect military personnel from 'venereal disease, including gonorrhoea' (Morton, 1976, p.120). Punitive measures were introduced which included the arrest, examination and treatment of 'loose' women. Women were thought to be the perpetrators. Those infected were forced to wear yellow clothing and were incarcerated in hospital wards known as canary wards.

16

The Victorian era

Queen Victoria reigned from 1837–1901 and this period is possibly one of the most discussed in terms of the history of sexuality. Victorian attitudes to sexuality dominated UK society's views until well into the middle of the twentieth century and many of the perspectives developed during this period are still evident today.

Key concepts during Victorian times were suppression and denial, and sexuality was controlled in the name of preservation and sanctity of the home and family. Double standards were rife. Codes of sexual behaviour, as life in general, were very different for different social classes and double standards between men and women prevailed. Women were expected to remain virgins until they married and the wife's responsibility was to look after the home and the needs of her husband. Women should be delicate, quiet and submissive. They were the objects of men's desires but should not enjoy sex or display sexual pleasure. One eminent London urologist even offered to 'solve the problem' by surgically removing the clitoris. Some Victorian women suffered because they, their husbands or their physicians were disturbed by their sexual desire and the assumption that women did not enjoy sex could become a self-fulfilling prophecy in that couples who held this view did not seek ways to enhance women's pleasure. Men were urged to marry late, usually around the age of 30 and were given tacit permission by society to sow wild oats, often with prostitutes or women from the lower classes.

On the surface Victorian society was repressive, dogmatic, arrogant and puritanical (Van Ooijen & Charnock, 1994). The sexual mood of the age was illustrated in Victorian environments and furniture, such as sofas designed to prevent people sitting closely together or piano legs which had to be draped in order not to suggest human legs. Language was also restricted, for example words such as breast, leg or thigh were discouraged, even when describing joints of meat. Euphemisms were common, for example prostitution was the 'social evil', gonorrhoea and syphilis were 'social diseases', birth control or sodomy were 'crimes against nature' and masturbation was 'self abuse'.

The double standards were not only between the classes and between men and women but also in the fact that sex was publicly denied whilst a secret culture of sex was thriving. Prostitution was rife throughout Victorian Britain and, by the mid nineteenth century, it was claimed that there were more brothels than schools (Van Ooijen & Charnock, 1994). Women turned to prostitution for a variety of reasons and particularly the social necessity of making a living in hard times. The stigma surrounding female sexual enjoyment, both inside and outside of relationships, had led to an increase in the use of female prostitutes but, as girlfriends increasingly 'gave way to the demands of their boyfriends' to have sex, prostitution began to decline around 1918 (Hyam, 1991). Male prostitution also existed but was seldom discussed. A small number of brothels specialised in men and boys, particularly linked to the military (Van Ooijen & Charnock, 1994).

Sexology in the Victorian era

Biological work predominated early writings on sexuality. In 1871 Charles Darwin suggested in *The Descent of Man, and Selection in Relation to Sex* that gender differences were rooted in sexual selection in that characteristics, such as peacocks' tail feathers, had developed to attract the opposite sex. Males were thus capable of attaining a higher eminence than women, 'whether requiring deep thought, reason or imagination, or merely the use of senses and hands'.

In *The Evolution of Sex* in 1889 two Scottish biologists, Patrick Geddes (1895–1932) and J. Arthur Thomson (1858–1935) maintained many of Darwin's assumptions concerning gender differences and pronounced that gender differences were simply reflections of the different metabolisms of the primary sex cells, the sperm and the egg. The sperm was 'catabolic' in that it was small, active and dissipated energy. The egg, by contrast, was 'anabolic' in that it was large, passive and energy conserving. They concluded that males were more active and variable; females were more passive and conservative.

In *Sex and Character*, 1903, Otto Weininger declared that

'the female is completely occupied and content with sexual matters [the spheres of begetting and of reproduction], whilst the male is interested in much else, in war and sport, in social affairs and feasting, in philosophy and science, in business and politics, in religion and art.'

(cited in Bland & Doan, 1998, p.25)

Paradoxically it was during the Victorian era that the debate about sexuality really developed and, against a backdrop of sexual denial and repression, scholars and scientists began to approach sexuality as a legitimate area for study.

The English physician Havelock Ellis (1859–1939) adopted two contradictory approaches in order to describe the roots of sexual behaviour and document its variations – biological determinism and cultural relativism (Weeks, 1989). Ellis's conclusions were both conservative and radical. He argued that female modesty was an inevitable by-product of male sexual aggressiveness, yet he stressed the erotic rights of women (Bland & Doan, 1998 p.13). Ellis compiled a series of volumes entitled *Studies in the Psychology of Sex*, published between 1897 and 1910. His interest in sexuality developed as a result of his personal experiences in that, as a young man, he experienced nocturnal emissions. The prevailing view of the con-sequences of such 'problems' included deafness, blindness, insanity or even death, and Ellis developed a lifelong interest in order to understand better his own and other people's sexuality. His sources included medical knowledge, anthropological findings and case histories, and his non-judgemental view of sexuality was illumi-nating, particularly considering the time at which he was writing. He contended that many sexual problems had psychological rather than physical causes; that sexuality behaviour starts at an early age and continues throughout the age range; that there are varying degrees of heterosexuality and homosexuality; that homosexuality was an inborn variation within the spectrum of sexuality rather than an aberration; that women experience sexual desire and often experience multiple orgasm; that orgasm in males and females is similar and that masturbation is common among both males and females.

Ellis found that many people suffered as a result of the pervading ignorance and suppression of sexuality. He advocated early sex education for boys and girls; acceptance of sexual behaviour in young children as a form of developmental self-exploration; sexual exploration for young couples before marriage; equal rights for women, especially for contraception and divorce; the right to private sexual behaviour by consenting adults of the same sex. Not surprisingly, Ellis's ideas were highly radical in Victorian times but it is interesting to note how many of the debates he raised are still current in British society in the twenty-first century.

The Viennese physician, Sigmund Freud (1856–1939) wrote *Three Essays on the Theory of Sexuality*, published in 1905. Freud's theory of personality proposed that humans are born with biologically-based sexual drives and that these are our prime motivating forces. Conflicts between sexuality and society become internalised as conflict between the *id* (the repository of biologically based drives or instincts) and the *ego* (representing reason and good sense). The ego seeks socially appropriate outlets for satisfying the basic drives which arise from the id. The moral conscience, the *superego*, sets high standards for behaviour. Freud introduced many new and controversial ideas about sexuality. His work is not without its critics but has exerted an enormous influence on modern science, culture and psychiatric medical practice.

As Bland and Doan (1998) contend, the theories of sexologists are not merely an academic matter; they affect how individuals conceive their sexual desires, impinge on the kinds of strategy developed by sexual reformers, and influence policy-makers in the drafting of social legislation.

Social reform in the early twentieth century

By the end of the nineteenth century, Britain had undergone major social changes, including rapid industrialisation, urbanisation and the disruption of old class patterns. The rise of the women's movement in the mid to late nineteenth century was challenging the existing role of women in society and claiming increased self-determination. Sexual behaviour was becoming inextricably linked with what Weeks (1989) describes as the politics of population. In the late nineteenth century, the larger size of working class families, with an average of four children, was seen as a major source of the perpetuation of poverty and ill health. Something like three of every five men presenting themselves for enlistment for the Boer War in 1898 were rejected as physically unfit. Sex was the key to the issue of population.

Gender roles and assumptions were changed fundamentally in the first two decades of the twentieth century by the women's suffrage movement and World War I. This period saw a significant reassessment of the role of women in society and within the family, and of female sexuality. There were active movements for sexual reform and greater availability of birth control. For example, Dora Black and Bertrand Russell, with whom she had an open marriage, founded a progressive school. Dora Russell wrote from the standpoint of a modern woman of the 1920s who knew from her own experience and that of friends and colleagues, that women were having affairs and that these did not have the deleterious effects ascribed to them by tradition. There was however still widespread caution among women about sex outside marriage as the consequences of an unwanted pregnancy could result in much hardship.

The avoidance of pregnancy by birth control methods had been discussed since the 1850s but was strongly rejected by the Catholic

Church and the medical establishment. Despite this the birthrate in Britain and most European nations had begun to decline from around 1870 and, among a variety of factors, it was becoming clear that the upper and middle classes were limiting births. Increasingly during the early twentieth century birth control was coming to be seen as having an essential role in the improvement of maternal health.

In 1918 Marie Stopes (1880–1958) wrote *Married Love*. This included both poetic accounts of women's nature and the potential of marriage and explicit accounts of the mechanics of sexual intercourse. Stopes opened the first of many subsequent clinics to offer birth control to married people. By the 1920s the middle classes were using birth control but many reformers wanted to reach the working classes. Some were influenced by eugenic fears about 'unfit' breeding, others by the need to improve maternal health and to prevent poverty and the possible disastrous consequences of abortion. In 1936 the Labour Party conference passed a resolution in favour of birth control advice in welfare centres but, largely due to Catholic opposition, it was 1940 before the Ministry of Health finally allowed advice for married women on medical grounds (Rowbotham, 1999).

Sexuality gradually began to receive increasing emphasis, for example the erotic passages in the early twentieth century writings of D. H. Lawrence, but by and large remained shrouded in ignorance and secrecy. Human sexuality was not widely taught in schools; few public forums featured erotica and few discussed sex openly. The most explicit sexual contact permitted in the films of the 1930s and 1940s was a discreet kiss (Weeks, 1989).

Homosexuality

Most works on the history of sex tend to concentrate on the major forms of sexual experience to the exclusion of the minority forms. This is not surprising given the importance of pair-bonding and reproduction in society. However, non-reproductive and non-heterosexual forms of sexuality expression, and indeed the control and regulation of them, are important aspects of social history. Attitudes towards homosexual behaviour, and the social and subjective meanings given to homosexuality, are culture-specific and have varied enormously across different cultures and through various historical periods (Weeks, 1989 p.97).

Male and female homosexuality have been viewed differently, particularly through the Christian influence and the perceived need

21

to protect procreative sex in marriage. Male homosexuality has been largely viewed as taboo, female homosexuality largely ignored. The duality of definition of homosexuality is significant:

> Homosexuality (from the Greek *homos*, meaning same [pronounced as in homologous]): feeling sexually attracted to people of the same gender. Homosexuality (from the Latin *homo*, meaning man [pronounced as in homo sapiens]): male sexually attracted to other males.
>
> (Collins English Dictionary (1991))

Regulation of homosexuality has mainly focused on male homosexual behaviour. In 1533 legislation passed by Henry VIII declared that all acts of sodomy were against nature and punishable by death. The death penalty continued on the statute books, formally at least, until 1861. In Britain the 1885 Criminal Law Act criminalised so-called acts of gross indecency between two men. Although lesbian behaviour was generally condemned, it was not explicitly recognised in legislation.

The trial of Oscar Wilde in the 1890s created what Weeks (1989, p.102) described as 'a labelling process of a most explicit kind drawing a clear border between acceptable and abhorrent behaviour' and also a public image for the 'homosexual', a term coming into use at that time. In the later decades of the nineteenth century however, there was clear evidence of the development of a new sense of identity among many homosexual individuals. The changing legal situation was intricately associated with the emergence of a 'medical model' of homosexuality and various explanations for homosexuality were offered, including hormonal, congenital, environmental or mental sickness. Would-be cures, such as hypnotism, chemical experimentation and aversion therapy, were attempted.

A male homosexual identity was thus beginning to emerge by the end of the nineteenth century but a recognisable lesbian identity was not apparent until the 1920s among professional women, and then only of public concern following a series of sensational scandals. Various reasons have been suggested for the low public profile of female homosexuality – the lack of acknowledgement of female sexuality generally, absence of legal regulation and consequent absence of public pillorying and the fact that overt sexual behaviour in homosexual females more closely resembles that of heterosexual females than that of homosexual males.

The debates about the possible causes, definitions and social regulation of homosexuality which took place particularly between the 1880s and 1930s have influenced subsequent thinking and Bland and Doan (1998, p.44) suggest that 'we are still struggling with their various legacies today'. The usefulness, however, of a binary distinction between hetero and homosexual is now strongly questioned.

> 'There is not a single homosexuality but homosexualities and there is no such thing as the homosexual or the heterosexual. Statements made about human beings on the basis of their sexual orientation must always be highly qualified'
> (Bell & Weinberg, 1978, p.23)

Conclusion

Throughout history, societies and cultures have developed their own standards for defining sexual values and the prevailing norms at any one time have determined what was regarded as normal/ abnormal, acceptable or unacceptable. Attitudes to sexuality and sexual behaviour have changed constantly through various periods of history. This chapter has offered glimpses of some of the extremes, while aiming to plot a general progression over time. Several issues highlighted in the chapter remain as influences and debates in contemporary society. The hypocrisy and double standards characteristic of the Victorian era, whereby sex was publicly denied while a secret sub-culture was thriving, periodically come to light, for example the abuse of young people by priests. The prejudice against same-gender relationships, and particularly between two men, witnessed in the late nineteenth century is also still in evidence. Examples of this can be seen in the repeated rejection of legislation to reduce the legal age of consent for gay men to that of heterosexuals, and the rejection of the repeal of section 28 of the Local Government Act 1988 banning local authorities from intentionally promoting sexuality.

British history, up until the mid twentieth century, had witnessed a fairly gradual evolution of societal attitudes concerning sexuality and sexual behaviour, but radical changes were about to take place.

References

Ahmed, R.A. (1991) Women in Egypt and the Sudan. In: L.L. Adler (ed.) *Women in Cross-Cultural Perspective*. Praeger, New York.

Bell, A.P. & Weinberg, M.S. (1978) *Homosexualities: A Study of Diversity among Men and Women*. Michell Beazley, London.

Bland, L. & Doan, L. (1998) *Sexology Uncensored: The Documents of Sexual Science*. Polity Press, Cambridge.

Branden, N. (1981) *The Psychology of Romantic Love*. Bantam, New York.

Ellis, H. (1936) *Studies in the Psychology of Sex*, Volume. 1. Random House, New York, p.464 (second edition). Cited in J. Weeks (1989) *Sex, Politics and Society: The regulation of sexuality since 1800*. London, Longman Group.

Foucault, M. (1979) *The History of Sexuality, Volume 1: An Introduction*. Allen Lane, London.

Gagnon, J.H. & Simon, W. (1973) *Sexual Conduct: The Social Sources of Human Sexuality*. Hutchinson, London.

Hyam, R. (1991) *Empire and Sexuality: The British Expeience*. Manchester University Press, Manchester.

Morton, R.S. (1976) Venereal diseases. In: *Encyclopaedia of Love and Sex*, pp.118–121. Marshall Cavendish, New York.

Nevid, J.S., Fichner-Rathus, I., Rathus, S.A. *et. al.* (1995) *Human Sexuality in a World of Diversity*, 2nd edition. Allyn & Bacon, Boston.

Nye, R.A. (1999) *Sexuality*. Oxford University Press, Oxford.

Padgug, R.A. (1979) On conceptualising sexuality in history', *Radical History Review*, **20**, Spring/Summer 1979, p.9.

Rowbotham, S. (1999) *A Century of Women: The History of Women in Britain and the United States*. Penguin, London.

Tannahill, R. (1980) *Sex in History*. Stein & Day, Briarcliffe Manor, NY.

Telushkin, J. (1991) *Jewish Literacy*. Morrow, New York.

Van Ooijen, E. & Charnock, A. (1994) *Sexuality and Patient Care: A guide for nurses and teachers*. Chapman & Hall, London.

Weeks, J. (1985) *Sexuality and its Discontents: Meanings, Myths and Modern Sexualities*. Routledge & Kegan Paul, London.

Weeks, J. (1989) *Sex, Politics and Society: The regulation of sexuality since 1800* (second edition). Longman Group, London.

2. *The Sexual Revolution*

Hazel Heath

No single event marked the onset of the sexual revolution but it lasted roughly from the mid 1950s to the mid 1970s. This was a period of profound social change in Britain, particularly in sexual attitudes and practices, driven by a combination of social, political, economic and scientific factors. Early 1950s life was in many respects more austere than it had been during World War II. For the British people, exhortations to duty and sacrifice were wearing thin and they were more than ready for the benefits of consumerism which sustained economic growth would soon bestow on them (Bruley, 1999). The time was also ripe for a rejection of the contradictions and absurdities of the puritanical codes which had prevailed during the Victorian era. The 1960s and 1970s saw major social upheaval, not only in sexual behaviour, but also in science, politics, fashion, music, art and cinema. In the early 1960s American folk singer Bob Dylan famously sang *The Times They are A-changin'*, and by the 1970s the so-called Woodstock generation, disheartened by commercialism and the Vietnam war, followed Timothy Leary's exhortation to tune in (to rock and pop music), turn on (to drugs) and drop out (of mainstream society) (Nevid *et al.*, 1995).

This chapter traces the development of a range of elements of sexuality and sexual behaviour during the period known as the sexual revolution. It considers concepts of sexuality in post-World War II Britain, and how these evolved during the 1960s. It highlights changing roles and the emergence of a youth culture characterised by greater liberation and permissiveness, as well as the appearance of counter-culture and protest movements. It concludes by describing the stream of legislation which was both influenced by, and in turn influenced, this historical period of unprecedented social change.

Post-war Britain

The early 1950s were a time of austerity and the shortages following World War II were making daily life difficult. Food rationing was even more severe than it had been in 1945; coal shortage cut train services; steel shortage closed factories, and housing shortage resulted in families living in prefabs (prefabricated buildings – flat-roofed boxes made of asbestos sheeting) often surrounded by bombsites, particularly in the major cities. In some respects, life was more bleak than during wartime. In addition, nuclear war was an ever-present dread (Lewis, 1978).

However, as the 1950s progressed an air of growing optimism developed, fed by continuing peace, rising living standards and the security of full employment. The 1951 Festival of Britain promised 'fun, fantasy and colour' and the outlook in Britain began to change (Bruley, 1999, p.130). Lewis (1978) described the 1950s as a major watershed in modern history, which moved from austerity to affluence. The decade brought advances in technology, greater international travel and increased mobility through the motor car. Lewis (1978) also highlighted the advent of sputniks, pop art, James Bond, Marilyn Monroe, Brigitte Bardot – new ideas, new sounds, new faces and new dilemmas, and observes that young people realigned their goals to fit the social change that surrounded them.

Sex in the 1950s

In the 1950s there was a dislike of 'making a fuss' about sex: mass observation found only about a third of people questioned thought a good sex life was essential to happiness (Rowbotham, 1999). Sex, it was felt, should not be made the be all and end all of life (Weeks, 1989). The 1950s was not a permissive era. In a questionnaire investigating English attitudes in 1950, Gorer found that 55% of men and 73% of women disapproved of women having sexual experience before marriage and about 50% disapproved of it for men. Gorer concluded, 'The high value put on virginity for both sexes is remarkable and, I should suspect, specifically English' (Gorer, 1950).

Despite the general impression of restraint, the double standards for men and women engaging in sexual activity continued – nice girls didn't but nice boys would if they could. Lewis (1978, p.43) writes that 'the would-be seducer of the 50s had to reckon with an armoury of unco-operative underwear which stood between him and his objective. The nylon stocking was still suspended from a constricting girdle of unyielding firmness, a fortification virtually impossible to bypass without active collusion and preferably plenty of time. The frustrated resorted to petting as a substitute'.

Female contraceptives in Britain were still kept out of sight but male condoms could be purchased, albeit furtively.

Changing roles

Men and women had experienced camaraderie in both the armed services and the hardships of life, including the bombings, at home. When they returned to family life and, after the post-war baby boom had settled, the small family became a permanent feature of British society. Expectations, however, were changing. One survey found that the quality men most desired in a wife was good housekeeping; the quality women most desired in a husband was understanding (Gorer (1950), cited in Rowbotham, 1999, p.304). Rowbotham observed that, '... with hindsight, it is easy to observe that the two sexes were not being reared for mutual comprehension'. Family life was idealised by the increasingly instant media, particularly television. 'The happy housewife beamed at the world from countless advertisements, looking out of her gadget-laden nest' (Lewis, 1978, p.46).

In addition, concepts of ideal family life and child rearing were changing. John Bowlby's *Child Care and the Growth of Love*, first published in 1953, argued the theory that the first five years of a child's life are crucial and that consistent maternal presence is the key, but both female and male family roles were changing. While men were still the major breadwinners they increasingly helped with household work and through the growing focus on natural childbirth increasingly became involved in the preparation for, and birth of, children. Dr Benjamin Spock's *Baby and Child Care* was first published in Britain in 1955. In contrast with previous orthodoxy of feeding by timetable and letting babies cry rather than spoiling them, Spock advised loving care and nurturing.

The fundamental changes experienced in male/female and family roles were not without repercussions. The Marriage Guidance Council (now Relate), which was then only prepared to counsel those whose sexual relations took place within marriage, was in its infancy in England as the 50s began. By the end of the

27

decade, however, its clientele had expanded by 30% and about one third of the cases were focused on relationships failing to meet expectations, particularly those of women. Twice as many women as men applied for help (Lewis, 1978 p.62).

The impact of changing expectations was also witnessed in Britain's divorce rate. By 1950, the pre-war rate had quadrupled from 8000 to 32,000 and the Royal Commission on Marriage and Divorce, appointed in 1951, was greatly alarmed by the trend. Its report, published in 1955, demanded less permissiveness and claimed that no-fault divorce by consent would lead to social disaster.

The trend for changing expectations and roles within families was reflected in the field of work. Both World Wars I and II had challenged the notion of men's work and women's work and, in 1946, the Royal Commission on Equal Pay argued for 'equal pay for commensurate work' for men and women but limited the applicability of this to lower grades in teaching, the civil service and local government. The recommendations were subject to fears that, if women's wages were raised significantly they might not view motherhood or unpaid work at home as attractive and that this could reduce the birthrate. The government of the day rejected the report on the grounds that it was inflationary.

By the 1950s, longer term trends in women's employment had asserted themselves. The most common types of work for female school leavers became secretarial and factory work (Bruley, 1999, p.121). However, the biggest change in women's employment in the post-war years, as revealed in the census returns, was the increasing number of married women workers. In 1931 the proportion of married women recorded at work was 10%, although this may have been an underestimation due to many women not declaring their earnings in official returns (Lewis, 1992, p.66). By 1951 it was 21%, and by 1972 it was 47% (Wilson, 1980, p.41). Despite the increasing numbers of married women workers, they experienced widespread discrimination in that they were often not considered as reliable or as committed as other employees, were not considered for promotion, and were excluded from sick pay schemes (Klein, 1965, p.24).

As the 1950s progressed, Britain became more affluent and cars, refrigerators, vacuum cleaners and other consumer goods became a part of everyday life for increasing numbers of the population. Women became increasingly indispensable as part of the workforce and their lives took on new perspectives as independent consumers, domestic companions and sexual partners. By the end of the decade, affluence had reached a level which prompted the then Prime Minister Harold Macmillan to say 'you've never had it so good'.

Mid-twentieth century sexology

Alfred Kinsey (1894–1939) was a zoologist at Indiana University. In 1938 Dr Kinsey had been asked to teach a course on marriage and, when researching for this, realised that little was known about sexual practices in American society. During the 1930s and 1940s he conducted the first large-scale studies of sexual behaviour. The research had some methodological flaws but his team conducted personal interviews with nearly 12,000 people across the USA and the results were published in two volumes: *Sexual Behavior in the Human Male* (1948) and *Sexual Behavior in the Human Female* (1953). The books became best sellers but, in a society unused to discussing sex openly, met with widespread criticism. His work had however revealed a major disparity between accepted attitudes towards sexual behaviour and actual sexual practice. Kinsey believed there was a need to study the human sexual response through direct scientific observation and was making plans to do so when he died in 1956.

William Masters, a physician, and Virginia Johnson, a researcher, studied changes which occur during sexual stimulation through direct and careful observation of nearly 700 men and women in laboratory conditions which was recorded on film. Their studies included masturbation and sexual intercourse and they treated these activities as a biological function. Their pioneering research was published in two books: *Human Sexual Response*, published in

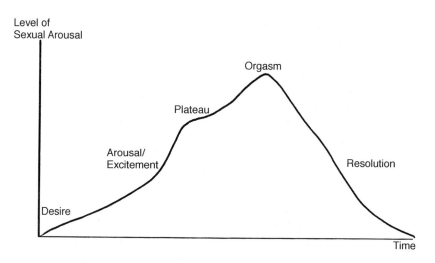

Fig. 2.1 Human Sexual Response Cycle (Masters & Johnson, 1966).

1966 and *Human Sexual Inadequacy*, 1970, and their work greatly enhanced understanding of the bodily changes which occur during sexual stimulation. A graphic representation of Masters and Johnson's work on the human sexual response cycle is shown in Fig. 2.1.

The work of Masters and Johnson, together with that of Helen Kaplan (1974), has considerably enhanced our understanding of the physiological and psychological aspects of sex and sexuality. Before this time, it was widely assumed that sexual dysfunction was largely psychogenic. It is now believed that organic factors may be involved in as many as 50% of cases. The work of the pioneers of this period still forms the basis of sex therapy programmes in the early twenty-first century.

The emergence of a youth culture

In the 1940s there was no accepted concept of a teenager but during the 1950s adolescent wages began to rise twice as fast as those of adults and the rapidly expanding consumer industries lost no time in producing goods specifically aimed at the new teenage market – clothes, records, cosmetics. The leisure market also opened up to young people with films and dance halls geared to teenagers (Bruley, 1999, p.135). One survey found that the youth of the post-war years was indulged as never before (Roberts, 1995).

Parents who had been through the war and possibly endured separation, bombing and post-war austerity sought, above all, to achieve a happy life for their children. They were noticeably less strict about enforcing discipline, although they did not abandon standards altogether. The youth of the 1950s and 1960s were more self-aware and more self-centred than any previous generation of young people. Feeling released from parental authority and with the freedom that money allows, they began to form distinct sub-cultures (Bruley, 1999, p.135). A definite teenage identity began to emerge with the Teddy Boys in the 1950s, followed by the mods and rockers of the early 1960s, the hippies and flower-power followers of the late 1960s and the skinheads and punks of the 1970s.

Elvis Presley made his first record in Memphis in 1953 and his fame spread but, reflecting the sexual controls of the era, he was only allowed to be shown on the television from the waist upwards to avoid his 'dangerous' pelvis from being seen. There were constant protests from Catholics, critics and guardians of public seemliness, and in Miami a charge of obscenity was levelled at his performance. In Britain, the record *Rock Around the Clock* was released by Bill Haley and the Comets in May 1955 and stayed at the top of the record charts for five weeks. The film of the same name, released the following year, was famed for causing riots in Britain. Fans ripped out cinema seats as they obstructed dancing and the disturbances were inflamed by the press who wrote about groups of Teddy Boys 'in an orgy of vandalism' (Lewis, 1978).

Liberation

During the 1950s and 1960s movements towards greater freedom were simultaneously taking place in many areas of life. Lewis (1978) suggested that the sexual liberation movement really began to flow in 1953, when Kinsey's report on *Female Sexuality* was published, but also with two other debuts – those of James Bond and *Playboy* magazine. 'The Puritan ethic was being replaced by the Hedonist ethic' (Lewis 1978, p.61). At a time when many women were learning about balancing conflicts between family roles and the lure of careers, the media of the time was promoting apparently con-flicting images of women – happy housewife or seductress.

One deciding factor in the 'liberation' of women was the facility to separate sex for procreation from sex for fun. Lewis (1978) observed:

'previous attempts to do this had always floundered on the fact that the fun usually resulted pretty soon in procreation but at this very time field trials of the contraceptive pill were taking place which would soon make the division practical and permanent for the first time in history' (p.62).

The oral contraceptive pill effectively ended the risk of unwanted pregnancy, permitting women to engage in sex for recreation, rather than for potential procreation. The pill was invented in 1952 and, once available, made a further baby boom unlikely. In 1958 the Church of England gave birth control its blessing under the name of family planning and the pill was introduced into Britain in 1961.

Counter-culture and protest

Within the 1950s climate of the Cold War, the H-bomb and the ever-present threat of nuclear devastation developed increasing pressure for disarmament. The National Council for the Abolition of Nuclear Weapon Tests was formed in 1957, after the H-bomb tests at Christmas Island and, in response to the Labour Party's refusal to support banning the bomb unilaterally, the Campaign for Nuclear

Disarmament was launched in January 1958. The momentum of protest was not limited to warfare.

> 'The anti-authoritarianism of direct action went into community politics, campaigns around pensioners' rights, protests about the draconian treatment of the homeless in hostels and libertarian education.'
>
> (Rowbotham, 1999, p.345)

Anti-establishment feelings were heightened in the early 1960s by the scandal involving John Profumo, then Minister of War, who had lied to Parliament in an attempt to cover up his involvement with Christine Keeler, who was simultaneously having an affair with a Russian spy who had been a military attaché at the embassy in London. The so-called moral laxity of the sexual intrigue was condemned as a product of the moral laxity of the age and the hypocrisy of the establishment was the target of the protests.

Protests were not limited to Britain. In the USA, passionate protests raged against the Vietnam war and racial discrimination. Student rebellions also took place in Europe in 1968. Hacker (1984, p.29) characterised the era as 'rebellion against the establishment and its old norms, and this launched a progressive erosion of the power of authorities such as parents and the church'. Bruley (1999, p.137) described how 'youth began to attack the values of the consumer society which had spawned them [and] dropping out became the thing to do'. Within this overall momentum, traditional prohibitions, including casual sex, group sex, 'free love' and erotic experiences heightened through drugs, were demolished in the tide of protest.

Permissiveness

During the 1960s the separation of sexual pleasure from procreation by more efficient means of birth control, alongside a greater understanding of sexual response from Masters and Johnson's work, and in particular of female sexuality, was highly liberating. It opened the doors to the pursuit of sexual pleasure for its own sake. At the same time society moved towards greater freedom, self-expression and liberation.

The media dealt more openly with sexual issues and this contributed to the breaking down of public and private barriers to what was acceptable. Books encouraged readers to explore their sexuality, commercialised sex became commonplace in major cities and sexually explicit film scenes became so commonplace that the film censorship rating system was introduced. In the increasingly pervasive visual media, sex became an aid to selling virtually anything and, in society as a whole, the range of what could be purchased, including sexual services, sex aids and recreational drugs, became increasingly visible.

Attitudes towards aspects of sexuality that had been condemned for generations, particularly by religious and establishment rulings, became increasingly relaxed. These included the taboos on birth control, abortion, divorce, premarital sex, extra-marital sex, cohabitation and homosexuality. Pornography was more readily available and 'girlie' magazines such as *Playboy* were accused of 'openly mass marketing masturbatory love' (Talese, 1980). There were backlashes against increasing permissiveness, such as Mary Whitehouse's campaign against those who had fallen prey to the exponents of the 'New Morality' (Whitehouse, 1971).

Some evidence of increasingly open attitudes to sex was offered from surveys in the USA. Kinsey's work in 1948 and 1953 suggested that, among the college-educated individuals interviewed in the 1940s, 27% of women and 49% of men had experienced premarital sexual intercourse by the age of 21. Surveys of college students in the 1970s report considerably higher incidences, ranging from 43 to 56% for females, and from 58 to 82% for males (Packard, 1970; Hunt, 1974). The greatest change in attitude towards premarital sex was seen in varying generations of women. In Hunt's (1974) national survey of 1400 individuals, 31% of those over the age of 55 (when completing the survey) said they had had premarital sexual intercourse, whereas 81% of those under 25 had done so.

Inferences on permissiveness can also be made from the use of the oral contraceptive pill, introduced into Britain in 1961. By 1964 half a million women were on the pill (Wellings *et al.*, 1994) and, as a result, the birthrate fell. In the early 1960s it had been rising, possibly because of increased sexual activity with less sure contraceptive methods. The number of births outside wedlock was rising, also possibly indicating that sexual activity was on the increase. This trend was not halted by the introduction of the pill. Contraceptive advice was initially only available for married women but, starting with the Brook Clinic in London in 1964, contraceptive advice was gradually made available to unmarried women. By 1969 rates of pill usage had increased sharply (Wellings *et al.*, 1994).

Permissiveness enabled individuals to separate sexual pleasure from any notion of commitment, but this was not without its risk or consequences.

Legislation

The stream of legislation from the late 1950s onwards reflected the pervasive and fundamental change taking place in British society and Rowbotham (1997) suggests that Parliament was responding to changing social attitudes, rather than initiating permissive policies. The 1959 Street Offences Act aimed to remove prostitutes from the streets but also led to court decisions which extended police jurisdiction over prostitutes into their own homes (Smart, 1981, p.51). It was subsequently illegal to solicit from doorways or windows. This was followed by the Obscene Publications Acts 1959 and 1964. The 1967 Sexual Offenders Act legalised homosexuality between consenting adults.

There had been movement towards legalising abortion during the 1950s, and the 1967 Medical Termination of Pregnancy Act, introduced by the Liberal, David Steel, legalised abortion if two doctors consented. The figures for abortions rose dramatically after 1967 but their accuracy must be questioned as undoubtedly there were also many thousands of backstreet abortions, posing a grave danger to women's health.

Unmarried mothers were no longer stigmatised quite so strongly as they had been previously and keeping a child, rather than handing over to an adoption agency, became increasingly acceptable (Lewis, 1992). The Family Planning Act enabled local authorities to provide advisory services on birth control. 1968 saw the implementation of the act abolishing censorship in the theatre. Under the 1969 Divorce reform law, divorce could be obtained on the grounds that a marriage had irretrievably broken down after a two-year separation if both parties wanted it, or five years if only one party sought the divorce. The Matrimonial Property Act secured the wife an equal share in family assets.

Conclusion

The historical period known as the sexual revolution saw rapid and unprecedented social changes. Many of the developments which took place during this time have left legacies which profoundly influence sexual attitudes, relationships and practices in the early twenty-first century. The most fundamental of these is in the societal, work and family roles of women and men. The era was characterised by rebellion against the establishment and its old norms, and this launched a progressive erosion of the power of authorities such as parents and the church. The so-called generation-gap was forged, and this was accentuated by the emergence of a distinct teenage identity and consumer market specifically aimed at young people. The consequences of the increased sexual freedom and permissiveness, viewed as progressive during the 1960s, have been far-reaching. The HIV/AIDS epidemic (discussed in Chapter 3) and the massive and socially problematic increase in teenage pregnancies are just two examples. Perhaps the major legacy of the sexual revolution is that we now experience 'two contrasting moralities' which, as Hacker (1984, p.29) suggests, appear to exist uneasily side by side – 'the new morality which encourages greater sexual activity at an ever younger age, and the old morality of denial that discourages dealing with it'.

References

Bowlby, J. (1953) *Child Care and the Growth of Love*. Penguin Books, Harmondsworth.

Bruley, S. (1999) *Women in Britain since 1900: Social History in Perspective*. Macmillan, Basingstoke.

Gorer, G. (1950) Exploring English Character, Criterion Books, New York. Cited in Lewis, P. (1978) *The 50s*. William Heinemann Limited, London.

Hacker, S.S. (1984) Students' questions about sexuality: implications for nurse educators. *Nurse Educator*, Winter 1984, 28–31

Hunt, M. (1974) Sexual Behaviour in the 1970s. Playboy Press, Chicago. Cited in Hilgard, E.R., Atkinson, R.L. & Atkinson R.C. (1979) *Introduction to Psychology*. Harcourt Brace Jovanovich Inc, New York.

Kaplan, H.S. (1974) *The New Sex Therapy*. Brunner/Mazel, New York.

Kinsey, A.C., Pomeray, W.B., Martin, C.E., & Gephard, P.H. (1948) *Sexual Behavior in the Human Male*. WB Saunders, Philadelphia.

Kinsey, A.C., Pomeray, W.B., Martin, C.E., & Gephard, P.H. (1953) *Sexual Behavior in the Human Female*. WB Saunders, Philadelphia.

Klein, V. (1965) *Britain's Married Women Workers*. Routledge & Kegan Paul, London.

Lewis, J. (1992) *Women in Britain since 1945*. Blackwell, Oxford.

Lewis, P. (1978) *The 50s*. William Heinemann Limited, London.

Masters, W. & Johnson, V. (1966) *Human Sexual Response*. Little Brown and Co., Boston.

Masters, W. & Johnson, V. (1970) *Human Sexual Inadequacy*. Little, Brown, Boston.

Nevid, J.S., Fichner-Rathus, I., Rathus, S.A., *et al.* (1995) *Human Sexuality in a World of Diversity* (second edition). Allyn & Bacon, Boston.

Packard, V. (1970) *The Sexual Wilderness: The Contemporary Upheaval in Male-female relationships*, David McKay Co. New York. Cited in E.R. Hilgard, R.L. Atkinson, & R.C. Atkinson (1979) *Introduction to Psychology*. Harcourt Brace Jovanovich Inc, New York.

Roberts, E. (1995) *Women and Families: An Oral History 1940–1970*. Blackwell, Oxford.

Rowbotham, S. (1999) *A Century of Women: The History of Women in Britain and the United States*. Penguin, London.

Smart, C. (1981) *Law and the Control of Women's Sexuality*. In: B. Hutter & G. Williams (eds). *Controlling Women: The Normal and the Deviant*. Croom Helm, London.

Talese, G. (1980) *Thy Neighbour's Wife: Sex in the World Today*, Collins, London.

Weeks, J. (1989) *Sex, Politics and Society: The regulation of sexuality since 1800* (second edition), Longman Group, London.

Wellings, K. *et al.* (1994) *Sexual Behaviour in Britain, the National Survey of Sexuality Attitudes and Lifestyles*. Blackwell, Oxford.

Whitehouse, M. (1971) *Who Does She Think She Is?* New English Library, London. Cited in Bruley, S. (1999) *Women in Britain since 1900: Social History in Perspective*. Macmillan, Basingstoke.

Wilson, E. (1980) *Only Halfway to Paradise: Women in Postwar Britain 1945–1968*. Tavistock, London.

3. Post HIV/AIDS: Emergence of a New Morality

Elizabeth Grigg

In 1981 the world was first alerted to a possible future Acquired Immune Deficiency Syndrome (AIDS) epidemic. During this time a multitude of social, sexual, psychological and medical questions have emerged around the experience of this complex, emotive and sensitive phenomenon. HIV, with all its implications, has proved to be more than just a disease.

The emergence of HIV and AIDS in the 1980s caused panic, blame and prejudice. It evoked moralistic behaviour akin to 'Victorianism' and a search for scapegoats (Western, 1999), which it found in black Africans, homosexuals, and intravenous drug users (IDUs). The legacy of HIV and AIDS has been widespread changes in attitudes and sexual behaviour; recent studies show that attitudes towards anything that is associated with sexuality are more conservative today than they were over a decade ago (Thompson, 1990).

It seems impossible to consider the impact of HIV and AIDS without consideration of human sexual behaviour (Dixon & Gordon, 1990). One of the unique characteristics of the virus is that it enables moralists to blame the victims of the disease for their illness. The label of HIV and AIDS continues to conjure up images of diverse sexual practices and malevolent human activities (Bunting, 1996; Hayter, 1996). HIV and AIDS continue to be associated with anal intercourse, drug misuse and promiscuity.

Added to this is the association of HIV and AIDS with loss and death, ethnicity and poverty, which are also some of the most vulnerable aspects of human life. They often arouse strong feelings and challenge deeply held values. The impact of HIV and AIDS may be the most critical condition that healthcare providers and populations have faced and will continue to face for many years to come.

Globally, the incidence of HIV continues to rise and carries on providing the world with major economic, physical, emotional, moral and social challenges.

This chapter traces the emergence of HIV and AIDS from the mid-1960s and describes the moralistic reactions to this. It offers an overview of current knowledge and available treatments. It also presents some global issues. The chapter concludes by highlighting some implications for nursing practice and the suggestion that the moralism, blame and prejudice which emerged in the 1980s still continue, even among health workers.

The emergence of HIV and AIDS

According to medical historians, HIV disease has possibly been within the human population for hundreds of years; however there was no evidence of illness in humans until the mid 1960s. Other medical historians argue that a benign form of HIV may have been infecting people for thousands of years and it was a modern mutation of the virus that actually triggered the present-day pandemic. They state that HIV probably lived as a relatively harmless virus in humans, but changes in human behaviour made it more virulent (Alcorn & Fieldhouse, 2000).

Even though poverty appears to have the greatest impact upon the spread of HIV, so-called AIDS made its dramatic initial entrance amongst the most socially mobile and well educated in Africa and among the affluent gay communities in the developed world. This is largely due to huge changes in many of the facets of society after the world wars, which are well documented. Increased mobility, the introduction of antibiotics and the contraceptive pill, less usage of barrier methods of contraception for sexual protection, and legal and sexual freedom all played a profound part in the sudden increase of the virus.

During the 1960s many gay men and lesbian women moved from small towns to larger cities to avoid prejudice and legal prohibition. For example, more than 50,000 gay men moved to San Francisco between 1969 and 1982. The economy and the social response that developed to service this migration was centred on uninhibited access to sexual pleasure. Arguably, increased sexual activity allowed the virus access to a variety of hosts. By natural selection the HIV was allowed to change and to mutate into a strong and life-threatening strain (Alcorn & Fieldhouse, 2000).

The emergence of AIDS in the 1980s caused panic, blame and prejudice. It took over from syphilis as a sexual plague. In the western world it evoked the same patterns of 'Victorianism' and moralistic behaviour in people as syphilis had done before antibiotics halted its spread. Society searched for scapegoats (Western, 1999) and found them in black Africans, homosexuals, and intravenous drug users. These groups were blamed for the spread of the disease. Black Africans were blamed for causing the disease in homosexuals in the first place; homosexuals were blamed for spreading HIV to haemophiliacs and IDUs; and IDUs were blamed for causing the disease in heterosexuals and children – the 'innocent victims'.

On 5 July 1981, the first five cases of AIDS were officially reported to a world unprepared for the epidemic to follow (World Health Organization (WHO), 1992). By the end of 1990 AIDS had caused over 20,000 deaths in Europe. On 1 July 1991, a total of 366,455 cases of AIDS had been reported from 162 countries. Of these 52,106 cases were in Europe. In 1995 the Centers for Disease Control and Prevention (CDCs) reported 548,102 AIDS cases in the United States and listed 343,000 deaths.

On World AIDS Day, 1 December 2000, the British media announced that there were over an estimated 34 million people worldwide infected with HIV, with the majority of them living in sub-Saharan Africa. The incidence in the United Kingdom (UK) amongst homosexual men and IDUs appears to have levelled off but the incidence in the UK for heterosexual exposure is still continuing to escalate. Worldwide, the Joint United Nations Programme on HIV and AIDS estimated that approximately 42% of people infected were reported to be women. Since the beginning of the global AIDS pandemic over 9 million children under the age of 15 years have lost their mothers. In sub-Saharan Africa 16 million people have died from AIDS. Disease associated with HIV now surpasses tuberculosis (TB) and malaria as the leading infectious disease and cause of death worldwide.

Predictions of the exact number of people infected with the virus are based upon the number of known infected individuals at the time of a study. The great majority of people only present for treatment when they have debilitating symptoms, and it is only then that they are tested and diagnosed as having an HIV related disease. Therefore any predictions are possibly conservative; the actual number of people with HIV or AIDS could be much higher. Some experts have stated that the known figures should be multiplied by ten for a more exact number of people actually infected.

In countries such as Africa, India, the Arab states, Thailand and so on, where there are very patchy and disparate public health services for people, it is virtually impossible to gather accurate statistics around the incidence of HIV infection.

Emergence of a new moralism

Arguably the last two decades of the twentieth century saw a return to the type of moralism found in the Victorian era (see Chapter 1). Western society had experienced a sexual revolution in the swinging sixties, with the advent of the contraceptive pill, the availability of penicillin and, in some countries, the acceptance of homosexuality (see Chapter 2).

All through history society has blamed the people who are on the fringes of society for disasters. Time and experience has not altered this phenomenon, it is just the catastrophe that changes. As Western (1999) states, disapproval hinders prevention. Censure stifles openness and stops people accessing help. HIV caused a marked disapproval of any diverse sexual behaviour that arguably led to covert, unprotected activities and an increase in the spread of HIV. Condemnation led to restrictive right wing legislation and an application of stigma to anything that did not reflect strong heterosexual family values. Homosexuality was seen as sinful. Sexuality education in schools in the UK reinforced these censures. Some schools were not even allowed to mention AIDS for fear that it might encourage children in learning about homosexuality.

HIV has affected the rich and famous and many prominent people have died from AIDS. It has maintained a high profile since it was first discovered and attracted greater funding from charities than many other diseases yet, despite all of this, it still remains an unacceptable disease to many – including nurses. Nurses, being part of society, have shared the prejudice, and even now some nurses are refusing to nurse anyone whom they perceive as displaying different sexual conduct to themselves. Some nursing institutions have refused to admit people with HIV. In 1990 a hospice in the south of England where some people dying of AIDS were being nursed was forced to close down. The relatives of the other patients were horrified that their loved ones were being nursed within the same environment as people who must have been gay.

Essentially all sexually transmissible infections are about sex and sex in this supposedly liberated and enlightened world is still a dirty word. As Hancock (1991, p.50) said:

'anything which has sexual overtones stimulates an unholy trinity of inhibition, hypocrisy and prejudice, all of which can and do have a detrimental effect on both prevention and care; this combined with ignorance produces a seemingly impenetrable barrier'.

Where are we now – an overview of present knowledge

HIVs belong to a group of viruses known as retroviruses; retroviruses, as parasites, need a host in order to survive. When retroviruses have few opportunities to meet new hosts they will preserve their present hosts in order to stay alive and reproduce. Killing off their host would be suicidal. If a strain of retrovirus such as HIV begins to encounter many new hosts, weaker hosts will allow the virus to breed unchecked and, by the process of natural selection, stronger mutations will develop. As a result of this the more robust mutations of the virus will inevitably kill their hosts.

According to Alcorn and Fieldhouse (2000), HIV-1 most likely mutated out of HIV-2. HIV-2 tends not to cause illness so quickly and is more difficult to transmit sexually and neonatally, whereas HIV-1 at present and without treatment can cause life-threatening opportunistic diseases; within months in some cases.

The physiology of HIV is well documented (Adler, 1995; Pratt, 1995; Alcorn & Fieldhouse, 2000). Retroviruses are responsible for many degenerative, immune deficient and malignant diseases. However they are very fragile and it is difficult for transmission to actually occur. Incidentally the hepatitis B virus and the hepatitis C virus, the latter of which is also a retrovirus for which there is no vaccination, pose a far greater risk of transmission than HIV. The risk of contracting hepatitis C from infected blood is estimated at about 3.5% compared to 0.3% for HIV. The risk of contracting hepatitis B from blood is approximately 30%.

The HIV retroviruses are unique and very complex. They are made up of elements that enable them to convert their particular genetic material into deoxyribonucleic acid (DNA), once they are inside the cell that they infect. The viral DNA then integrates with the host cell DNA and creates a continuing infection.

After humans contract the virus there is a period where the virus is non-active. After a period of weeks, or in some cases months, the infected cell is stimulated into manufacturing more viruses copied into their original form. The host cell thus acts as a factory producing copies of the retrovirus that originally infected it. When enough viruses have been produced they burst out of the host cell to infect further cells in the body (Pratt, 1995).

HIVs have a special attraction to the T 'helper' cells or macrophages. However there are other cells in the body which contain the properties that HIV locks onto and enters. For example, HIV may directly affect the central nervous system (CNS) and therefore the brain and spinal cord.

At the moment only three HIVs have been specified: HIV-1, HIV-2 and HIV-1-0. HIV antibody tests will detect HIV-1 and HIV-2 but not HIV-1-0 (Pratt, 1995). However, after a person is infected with HIV, at replication each generation of the virus changes, or mutates, which makes exact testing, vaccination and anti-retroviral treatment extremely complex. At present eight major sub-types of HIV-1 and one major sub-type of HIV-2 have been identified (Alcorn & Fieldhouse, 2000). As with hepatitis C there is no vaccination available for any of these viruses.

Individuals infected with the viruses react in different ways. Damage to the T cells, and hence to the immune system, may result in some people becoming ill with opportunistic infections within weeks whilst others may take years to develop any of the symptoms associated with an AIDS defining condition.

Since the introduction of complex anti-retroviral therapies and sophisticated prophylactic care many individuals, having been diagnosed with AIDS, may now overcome their symptoms. Arguably they could be said to have reverted back to 'just having HIV'. To some people being given the diagnosis of AIDS seems like a death sentence; final, psychologically damaging and offering no hope, whereas a diagnosis of infection or disease associated with HIV gives a more positive message – a message that associated infection can be conquered.

AIDS (or HIV disease)

When the immune system breaks down people become vulnerable to opportunistic infections, some of which can be fatal (Pratt, 1995). Most people who develop symptoms associated with their HIV will present with one or more opportunistic infections at the same time. The commonest disease seen, as well as being the most frequent cause of death, is pneumocystis carinii pneumonia (PCP). Interestingly PCP was thought to have been a protozoan induced opportunistic infection, but more recent research has shown that PCP is induced by fungal infection (Alcorn & Fieldhouse, 2000).

If the body is immuno-compromised, other opportunistic infections arise. Normal body pathogens such as viruses, bacteria, fungi and protozoa will present as infections. For example, infections such as genital or oral sores caused by the herpes simplex virus and cytomegolavirus retinitis, which is also caused by the herpes virus, may present. Incidentally the herpes simplex virus is present in one in four people and will often lie dormant until a person becomes immuno-compromised. Any ulcer or sore, including those caused by a sexually transmittable infection (STI), provides a route for HIV infection to occur. Epidemiological evidence also points to other STIs assisting HIV infection, although the mechanism through which this takes place is not clear. Tuberculosis (TB) is also linked closely with HIV infection, especially in Russia, where draconian laws do little to assist people holistically (Alcorn & Fieldhouse, 2000).

In the developed world the prophylactic care for most opportunistic infections is now very efficient. Many physicians will prescribe antibiotics or treatment before the onset of an infection according to an individual's CD4 count. Many people with HIV have their CD4 count monitored every three months. Some even have a check once a month. This enables a measurement of the immune status, or T cells, and provides a guide as to when opportunistic infections are likely to occur. The lower the CD4 count the fewer T 'helper' cells are present. The immune system is therefore compromised and there will be a greater chance of an individual with HIV acquiring an opportunistic infection.

Use of 'combination therapy', anti-HIV drugs or anti-retroviral treatment

As well as recommending regular checks on an individual's CD4 count, medical personnel will also propose regular viral load counts to determine the amount of virus present in the blood and indicate when treatment with anti-retroviral drugs could begin. It is argued that the lower the viral load is kept the better the prognosis will be.

Currently the British HIV Association (BHIVA) advocates that treatment should always be offered to people within six months to nine months of contracting HIV. However, many people are only diagnosed after they present with symptoms, which could in fact be much later. At present there is no conclusive evidence to suggest the best time to start anti-viral therapy and therefore the BHIVA advise starting it when the benefits of treatment outweigh the benefits of not starting treatment, that is, if the CD4 count is 350 cells regardless of the viral load, if the CD4 count is above 350 cells but falling rapidly and if the viral load is above 30,000 at any CD4 count (Alcorn & Fieldhouse, 2000).

Anti-retroviral therapies involve a combination of drugs that suppress the replication of HIV. Different anti-virals attack the various stages of the HIV life cycle. There appear to be six stages to HIV replication (Alcorn & Fieldhouse, 2000). At present drugs that work on the first stage, when fusion takes place, are about to enter clinical trials. Zidovudine (AZT) and other non-nucleoside analogues target the second stage. At present there is also no clear evidence as to which combinations of drugs should be commenced initially.

Anti-retroviral therapy is problematic. First, there are major side effects for some people, problems of compliance for others and huge cost and inequality implications involved. Second, and perhaps more important than all the above is the complacency that treatment and possible cure brings with it. The general public hears messages that treatment is advancing and that soon there will be a 'cure':

> 'People are saying that instead of taking six pills rigidly four times a day [the present anti-retroviral treatment] soon there will be only one pill once a day to take ... people do not take precautions because of this ... they are having sex all over the place ... nothing has changed.'
> (Andy Andrews (Body Positive Somerset) who was diagnosed with HIV in 1990) 1 January, 2001

Third, there is also an increasing awareness amongst researchers of the issue of HIV mutation in the face of anti-retroviral therapy, causing strains of HIV to become drug resistant through natural selection (Alcorn & Fieldhouse, 2000). It is argued that transmission of certain drug resistant HIVs could lead to strains of HIV combining to produce a type of HIV which could be multi-drug resistant and therefore far more treacherous and prolific.

But fourth, and as mentioned above, because of advances in all forms of treatment, many people are living longer with their virus. The psychological impact of this is vast. As Andy Andrews (2001) states:

> 'Ten years ago I was given a death sentence and told that I had only months to live. I prepared for death and waited to die. Four years later it had not happened and so I began to live again. The psychological implications of this are a "minefield". I have learnt to live with this thing inside me ... but it has taken me a long time to come to terms with it.'

Poverty, sex and HIV

In the developed world, tax cuts for the wealthy have meant that there is less to spend upon health and welfare provision for the poor. In the developing world, countries have had to focus upon their international debts rather than upon the provision of public health services. Poverty limits access to health care. Although it continues to be recognised that the poorest in society have the poorest health status, little is done to address it (Alcorn & Fieldhouse, 2000).

Poverty also forces people to sell sex for survival, rendering many of the most vulnerable underprivileged in society at high risk of contracting HIV and other STIs. In developed countries these people may be able to access treatment but in the developing world there is little hope that people with HIV are able to benefit from anti-retroviral treatments, not only because of cost issues but also because of the lack of adequate medical infrastructures.

Women with HIV, and especially women in poverty with HIV, appear to suffer from stigma to a far greater extent than men. Throughout history women have been socially constructed as deviant and of a lower status than men. Historically, women have taken the blame for wars, famine and disease (Bunting, 1996). Bunting (1996) describes studies that have shown that men and women respond very differently to a diagnosis of HIV. Some gay men are proud of the way they have contracted their infection – through rough sex and multiple partners; whereas most women are ashamed and terrified.

Women and HIV

Alcorn and Fieldhouse (2000) claim that in every day in 1999 at least 6300 women in the world became HIV positive. In the same year 3287 women died of HIV diseases. In sub-Saharan Africa there are now 12 women to every 10 men infected with the virus. Discrimination against women with HIV has a long history. Women in Africa, Thailand and women of African and Hispanic descent in America have been automatically blamed for being the drug users and the prostitutes causing the infection in their men. Women were excluded from drug trials until very recently. Bunting (1996) claims that the reason why pregnant women especially are now included in research is because of the potential benefit to the fetus rather than to the woman.

In most parts of the world HIV is increasing faster amongst

women than amongst men. The reasons are multiple and complex and involve many physiological, biological, social and psychological factors.

Biologically and physiologically it is easier for women to contract HIV from men, either through vaginal or anal intercourse, than it is vice versa. Women in poverty are often very young when they commence sexual intercourse for whatever reason. Their vaginal walls and hymen will therefore be thin and susceptible to damage. Coercive sex is also a common feature of many women's lives. Some research has estimated that 30% of women in South Africa had been coerced into their first sexual intercourse with 11% of these women stating that they had been raped (Alcorn & Fieldhouse, 2000).

Some cultures still continue to practice infibulation on women and to use agents to tighten or dry the vagina for male pleasure. The operation of infibulation itself is often covert and illegal and lends itself to poor operating practice and therefore to a high risk of blood contamination. Agents that cause tightening of the vagina are often abrasive and may cause bleeding, also inducing a high risk of HIV transmission. Alcorn and Fieldhouse (2000) state that 25% of heterosexuals practise anal intercourse – a fact hardly ever addressed. In some cultures women may engage in anal sex to preserve their virginity.

There are many diverse social and psychological factors to consider. The low status of women in nearly all societies makes them psychologically and socially vulnerable. Issues such as the conspiracy of silence for women around sex make it impossible for some women to seek out information. Globally, many more women than men remain illiterate. Women's low self-esteem in the face of men does not allow them the confidence to negotiate safer sexual practices – even if they are aware of them. Many women fear that requesting a partner to wear a condom is questioning his fidelity and may provoke violence. It is easier to remain accepting and silent.

In most societies it is the male who chooses the female and many older men will choose younger women to have sexual intercourse with. This increases the risk to women who have intercourse with men with a longer sexual history than they do. The economic status of many women means that they may have few alternatives. They can remain in a coercive relationship where they at least have the chance of a secure social and economic position or leave it to exchange sex for money, drugs or goods.

In Britain many women maintain that they are aware of the risk of HIV but are unaware that it could apply to them. As Alcorn and

Fieldhouse (2000) assert, the constant discussions around hetero-sexual AIDS fail to delineate the differences between women and men and risk behaviours. Women and men place different meanings on sexual activity. Sexuality remains more acceptable in both gay and straight men. As Bunting (1996) discusses, since the Stonewall rebellion in 1969, gay men have developed pride in their sexual orientation and many have celebrated this pride in having sex with many male partners. Straight men have also been proud of their own high levels of sexual activity and as Bunting (1996) states male sexual promiscuity is accepted and revered; whereas female sexual promiscuity continues to be considered as deviant and intolerable.

Nursing care and HIV

There has been extensive research around nurses' attitudes towards caring for people with HIV illnesses (Grigg, 1994; Hayter, 1996; Grigg, 1997; Ventura, 1999) to name but a few. All of these studies show that when nurses are faced with caring for people with these conditions they show feelings of confusion, prejudice, anxiety, fear and concern. The studies illustrate that the confusion that some nurses experience results from their individual opinions and attitudes. These stem from their value systems around the concept of HIV as a disease of fault and consequently the result of diverse sexual and behavioural practices.

In the early 1990s the Department of Health (DoH) and the English National Board (ENB) set up structures and training packages to address these issues. An attempt was made to introduce sexuality education into all healthcare programmes, to deal with attitudes, knowledge, stigma and prejudice. However financial constraints and the changing political climate, which influences the purchase of healthcare education, have stifled this initiative. In Britain HIV and AIDS have not reached the epidemic proportions that were predicted and funding has shifted to other priorities.

Perhaps reassuringly, Ventura's (1999) survey shows that nurses are more confident in dealing with the nursing care of people with HIV disease, in terms of infection control and related issues, than they were at the beginning of the 1990s. However her study also reflects those findings of the research that was completed at the outset of the HIV panic. Nurses remain less than confident, and indeed judgmental, when dealing with the ethical, psychological and moral matters that surround people with HIV disease.

The psychological implications of HIV

Lavery (2000) states that in her work as a clinical nurse specialist in HIV/AIDS she is witnessing many people with HIV living longer and that the incidence and complexity of the psychological needs of her clients are enormous. She continues that, perhaps more than ever before, there is an increasing need to raise awareness of the psychological needs of this client group and to ensure that skilled mental health input is available.

It is vital that this psychological support is provided from the very first moment that someone with concerns about their HIV status accesses health care services. It is most likely that it will be a nurse who provides this initial contact during the antibody test for the virus. Whether the test is positive or negative, support must be provided.

Serological tests for HIV are not always conclusive and may even become less accurate as the virus becomes more complicated by mutation. As well as this, some people may not have developed antibodies but have sought a test before sero-conversion has had time to take place. Some people may never produce adequately defining antibodies, although this is rare. The counselling skills of nurses are central to how these situations are managed. But nurses need support in order to deal with these complex and emotional matters. The practical constraints that nurses face are often under-estimated. Nurses, being part of society, are no more immune from panic, fear and prejudice than any other group in society (Grigg, 1994).

Conclusion

Attitudes to sexually transmitted infections have changed throughout history, but the occurrence of HIV provoked fear, prejudice and a backlash akin to the moralism of the Victorian era. This backlash has left its legacy and attitudes towards anything associated with sexuality are more conservative today than in 1980 (Thompson, 1990).

As more treatments become available and the life expectancy of people with HIV in the developed world becomes greater, it is critical for nurses and healthcare workers to focus upon the quality of life that they can promote for individuals. But healthcare workers must not lose sight of the global impact of HIV. Nurses and healthcare workers are key in providing hope for individuals and their loved ones who are affected by the virus wherever they are.

HIV and AIDS continue to be a huge challenge for nursing. The disease and all of its accompanying effects encompass some of the most controversial and emotional issues that nursing and health care have had to, and continue, to face. In order for nurses to feel comfortable about meeting the needs of people with this condition, they must begin with themselves and examine their own feelings about sex and sexuality, drugs and their misuse, and their feelings about death and dying.

Although HIV/AIDS has maintained a high profile and has attracted greater funding from charities than many other diseases, it still remains an unacceptable disease to many, including nurses. This is illustrated in a statement from a nurse tutor:

> '... frankly I have no sympathy with homosexuals who contract the disease. This is because it has been contracted through performing an unnatural act – a biological fact. Therefore while nurses have a duty to care for the sick we must also recognise that it is "self-inflicted" in the truest sense of the term, and need not have arisen in the first place. What makes AIDS more horrific is that a stranger's perverse sexual actions can harm totally unknown innocents.'
>
> (Sim, 1992, p.572)

This statement, although made nearly a decade ago, reflects society's attitude towards the consequences of a so-called diverse human sexual act. It reflects the blame, the shame and the stigma that have always surrounded sexually transmitted infections. Disapproving attitudes towards anything that carries a sexual connotation results in secrecy. Additionally, increasing infection and treatment brings about resistance and viral mutation that will contine to provide a challenge for care and for cure.

References

Adler, A. (1995) *ABC of AIDS* (third edition). BMJ Publications, London.

Alcorn, K. & Fieldhouse, R. (2000) *AIDS Reference Manual*. NAM Publications, London.

Andrews, A. (2001) from a conversation, 1 January.

Bunting, S. (1996) Sources of stigma associated with women with HIV. *Advances in Nursing Science*, **19**, 2, 64–73.

Dixon, H. & Gordon, P. (1990) *A Handbook for Those Involved in Training on HIV/AIDS*. Family Planning Association, London.

Grigg, E. (1994) *The value that nurses put on sexuality education*. MA Thesis, School Of Education And Health Studies. South Bank University, London.

Grigg, E. (1997) *A situational analysis of an HIV/AIDS clinical area. Journal of Clinical Nursing,* **6**, 1, 35–41.

Hancock, C. (1991) The challenge for nurses. *Nursing Standard,* 16 January, **5**, 17.

Hayter, M. (1996) Is non-judgmental care possible in the context of nurses' attitudes to patients' sexuality? *Journal Of Advanced Nursing,* **24**, 4, 662–6.

Lavery, A. (ed.) (2000) Newsletter, November. The HIV & Mental Health Nurses Special Interest Group, East Yorkshire.

Pratt, R. (1995) *AIDS: A Strategy For Nursing Care.* Edward Arnold, London.

Sim, J. (1992) AIDS, nursing and occupational risk: an ethical analysis. *Journal of Advanced Nursing,* Jan., **17**, 569–75.

Thompson, J. (1990) Sexuality: the adolescent and cancer. *Nursing Standard,* 6 June, **4**, 37, 26–49.

Ventura, M.J. (1999) The realities of HIV/ AIDS. *Research Nurse,* **62**, 4, 26–31.

Western, A. (1999) *Sexually Transmitted Infections.* NT Books, London.

4. *Nursing as a Sexualised Occupation*

Isabel White

The first three chapters of this book considered the historical influences upon sexuality as manifest within society, in particular those which have had lasting influences on personal beliefs, values and sexual expression in contemporary Britain. The way in which sexuality as a concept is constructed by nurses and other healthcare professionals, both individually and collectively, is not only influenced by such beliefs and values. It is also influenced by the perspectives of clients, patients, relatives and by popular media images of nurses, patients, illness, disability, sex and sexuality.

Crucially such value-sets frequently determine whether or not a nurse (or their patient/client) considers sexual issues relevant solely when an illness and its treatment directly affect sexual function or reproductive capacity (White, 1994). Other factors influencing the extent to which nurses address sexual issues in their practice include the possession of a satisfactory knowledge base (Webb, 1988), the nature of sexual health content taught within nurse education programmes (Bernhard & Dan, 1986; Pryce, 1991) and whether or not the discussion of such matters evokes embarrassment for the nurse (Lewis & Bor, 1994).

While the chapters in Part 3 of this book discuss the impact of specific nursing contexts and client need upon the nature of sexuality within practice, this chapter explores some of the hidden cultural and organisational influences upon individual practice. It also exposes the challenge inherent in establishing appropriate professional relationships and boundaries when sexuality is viewed as an integral, and at times problematic, facet of contemporary nursing practice.

Portrayal of sexuality in nursing literature and education

An historical analysis of nursing texts reveals, not surprisingly, that attitudes towards sexuality in the nurse–patient relationship reflect the prevailing norms and values of society at the time of publication (Bullough & Seidl, 1987). At the turn of the century nursing, and women's, apparent denial and repression of anything sexual was exemplified by Hampton-Robb's textbook published in 1907. This general text for nurses explicitly avoided mention of the genitalia when performing personal hygiene for patients and thus directed nurses to wash '. . . the surfaces between the thighs'. As early as 1913 nurses were playing a role in sex education of the time in warning people about the dangers of 'self-abuse' (masturbation) and of the need for 'sexual restraint' in the promotion of social hygiene (Bullough & Seidl, 1987).

Throughout the 1960s and 1970s sexuality began to be promoted within nursing education in relation to the biology of human reproduction. The growing influence of the feminist movement and increased emphasis upon an emergent female sexuality through the works of Kinsey *et al.* (1953), Masters and Johnson (1966) and Hite (1976) began to influence the teaching of sexuality within the nursing curriculum, in the United States at least (Bullough & Seidl, 1987). However, despite such progress, even as late as the 1970s nursing texts contained strong moralistic undertones, citing '. . . sex as a major causal factor of social ills such as divorce and child abuse' (Bullough & Seidl, 1987).

The explicit inclusion of sexuality within some theories of nursing, for example those of Johnson, Watson, Roy and Roper, and Logan and Tierney, may have assisted in making it a concept of legitimate concern to the discipline of nursing. However, to date there have been only limited attempts to provide a considered analysis of the concept within health care or nursing practice. Nor has there been an adequate exploration of the implications of raising the profile of sexual health within mainstream care delivery from either a theoretical or clinical perspective within the field of general nursing (Savage, 1989). American and British nurse literature from 1980 onwards reveals increasing interest in and concern about the professional nursing response to sexual issues within practice.

An analysis of 350 written responses from American graduate and undergraduate nursing students regarding sexuality in nursing, identified seven areas of concern in relation to human sexuality within nursing practice (Hacker, 1984). These were sexual conflict within the nursing role (harassment and difficult personal feelings), sex and its relationship within ill health or disability, contraception, homosexuality, adolescent sexuality and teenage pregnancy and the sexual needs of 'special' groups such as older people, those experiencing mental illness and people with learning difficulties.

The underlying theme that pervaded all questions raised by students was that of achieving some degree of 'comfort' for nurses in the discussion of sexuality (Hacker, 1984). Regrettably, the analysis presented did not include any explanation as to why, among other issues raised, the students classified older people as a 'special group' in relation to sexuality. This may suggest the prevalence of ageist assumptions and negative stereotyping of older people as found in the theoretical and research literature reviewed in Chapter 9.

In contemporary American and British nurse education, many nursing departments continue to teach sexuality within or in conjunction with obstetric, gynaecological or genito-urinary pathology and course content (Bernhard & Dan, 1986; Pryce, 1991). Bernhard and Dan (1986) would suggest that such an approach reinforces traditional attitudes to sexual behaviour and places undue emphasis on the relatively narrow association between sexuality and reproduction. Clearly while sexuality remains framed within the apparently 'more respectable' context of reproduction, or within the study of specific body systems, more diverse and less traditional definitions of sexuality remain on the margins of nursing awareness and thus of both professional acceptability and response.

Sexual stereotyping

Sexual stereotyping arguably remains a dominant controlling and detrimental influence upon the role definition, role conduct and role evolution of both male and female nurses within contemporary healthcare practice.

While much has been written about the image of nursing, Kalisch and Kalisch (1982a, b, c) were the first authors to formally study the relationship between the contemporary role of the nurse and the values that American society held about the profession, as expressed subliminally through the popular media of novels, films and television.

The results of a content analysis of 670 nurse and 466 doctor characters portrayed in novels, films, and prime-time television over the years 1920–1980 pointed to a steady decline in the image of nurses portrayed in the mass media, while that of the doctor remained consistently high or actually showed improvement (Kalisch & Kalisch, 1986).

Many would agree that little has changed in the current portrayal of nursing in British society since this research was conducted. There remains an urgent need to reduce the negative impact of persistent and restrictive gender role stereotypes on the actual and potential contribution of nurses within health care in general and sexual health care more specifically.

While the origins of the stereotype of the sexually permissive female nurse may be explored from a variety of perspectives (Lawler, 1991; Porter, 1992) a sociological analysis would suggest that this particular stereotype is a phenomenon of recent years (Kalisch & Kalisch, 1982a, b, c; Fiedler, 1988; Hunter, 1988; Aber & Hawkins, 1992).

Prior to the 1960s, the media portrayal of nurses was that of '...chaste young women'. However, the dawn of an era marked by so-called sexual liberation led to female nurses being increasingly viewed as the '...promiscuous playthings of their male medical colleagues' (Porter, 1992, p.521). Porter's rationale as to why nurses are singled out, more than any other female occupational group, as the recipients of sexual innuendo, jokes and stereotyping relates to the fact that much of nursing work involves intimate physical contact with people's bodies. This will be explored in some detail in Chapter 5.

Earlier work related to the image of nursing by Fagin and Diers (1984) suggested that as well as representing many other facets of the traditional female role in what remains predominantly a patriarchal society, nursing can also be seen as a metaphor for sex:

> '...having seen and touched the bodies of strangers, nurses are perceived as willing and able sexual partners. Knowing and experienced they, unlike prostitutes, are thought to be safe: a quality suggested by the cleanliness of their white uniforms and their professional aplomb.'
>
> (Fagin & Diers, 1984, p.17)

Men in nursing still constitute a minority of healthcare professionals employed in direct patient care, particularly in general nursing, from which the sexual stereotype of the gay male nurse appears to emanate. One explanation for the emergence of such a stereotype is the gendered division of labour in health care (Davies, 1995) where nursing is strongly identified as a metaphor for all things feminine and the natural assumption may be that men in nursing must therefore possess a predominance of female attributes. Evans (1997) further develops this argument in asserting that the '... labelling of men nurses as odd or homosexual can also be interpreted as a social control mechanism which re-defines nursing as women's work...' (p.228). It is therefore no surprise that men in nursing predominate in specialities and posts that appear more congruent with a masculine gender role stereotype in both behaviour and non-traditional dress such as psychiatry, intensive care, accident and emergency or research, educational and managerial posts.

An interesting observation is that the stereotype of the gay male nurse does not appear to have been exploited by the popular media to the same extent, or explored through the nursing literature regarding nursing image. Is the privilege of a patriarchal society and its healthcare system operating successfully to protect men in nursing from the professional image distortion only deemed appropriate for its female subordinates?

The experience and contribution of lesbian nurses is even more invisible in the public discourse regarding nursing image, with mainstream nursing literature failing to acknowledge their existence, reinforcing again the invisibility of female sexualities outwith the context of their response to a masculine counterpart.

The apparent invisibility of anything sexual within nursing work was more recently exemplified in Lawler's study of 'body work' in nursing (1991). She initially omitted questions specifically related to sexuality from the interview schedule of her ethnographic study of the concept of the body and 'body work' in nursing. It was only during the conduct of interviews with nurses, when spontaneous mention of issues relating to sexuality and the body occurred, that Lawler included sexuality as a central theme in her analysis of the concept of 'embodied existence'.

Lawler (1991) provided an in-depth analysis of the problems created for an occupation such as nursing in its care of the 'sexualised body'. Despite the fact that repeated, yet non-sexual, touch is a fundamental aspect of nursing care, much of nurses' work is heavily inscribed with sexual meaning. This necessitates the creation of ritualised coping strategies whereby nurses attempt to make this aspect of their work manageable and acceptable for all parties concerned through the reduction of both personal and patient embarrassment (Lawler, 1991).

The desire to avoid confirmation of sexist and derogatory imagery relating to the professional role of the nurse and to their role (predominantly) as women in wider society, may serve to control or suppress the sexuality inherent in nursing practice to the point of retarding its appropriate acknowledgement, research and development. What is clear is that society and its popular media culture remain fascinated by the sexual imagery inherent to healthcare professionals and their gendered provision of intimate care within the emotionally charged context of illness, vulnerability and loss.

Sources of prejudice in the nurse–patient relationship

As discussed in the first three chapters of this book, the issue of sexuality is one that normally engenders firmly held individual beliefs and values that have been formed through child rearing and socialisation processes.

The United Kingdom Central Council (UKCC, 1992) code of professional conduct for nurses places emphasis on the practitioner's ability to:

> '...recognise and respect the uniqueness and dignity of each patient and client, and respond to their need for care, irrespective of their ethnic origin, religious beliefs, personal attributes, the nature of their health problems or any other factor.'
>
> (UKCC, 1992: clause 7)

Inherent to the conduct of such professional practice is the nurse's ability to avoid the influence of individual beliefs on the delivery of care. However as Hayter (1996) remarks, this stance of professional neutrality appears to oversimplify the complex issues that arise in contemporary clinical practice. He cites a number of studies from the mid 1980s and early 1990s (Douglas, 1985; Webb, 1988; Kautz *et al.*, 1990) that demonstrate the negative attitudes expressed by nurses in relation to the sexual orientation of their patients. Furthermore, these nurses also expressed a high level of anxiety related to their perceived inability to discuss sexual matters with these clients, or to incorporate sexuality within care delivery. The majority of these studies emerged during the years when the impact of AIDS and HIV infection was at its height and one could be complacent in believing that it was ignorance and fear of contracting this infection that led to prejudicial care. However, as Hayter (1996) remarks, it could also be argued that the advent of HIV merely served to legitimise negative attitudes of nurses towards homosexual patients rather than to create them. Bancroft's (1989) work in the field of psychosexual medicine supports this view, stating that almost every society continues to hold negative attitudes towards homosexuality. As nurses are also part of a wider society it is not surprising that such mores and values influence them in the context of care delivery.

Identification of the precise extent to which such attitudes affect the quality and nature of care delivery requires further exploration within the research literature. While nurses appear to believe that holding negative attitudes need not adversely affect care unless verbalised or acted upon with patients, this view is not supported by the literature (Johnson & Webb, 1995). Seminal work on the impact of stigma (Goffman, 1968) and that of Sundeen *et al.* (1989) on the concept of exclusion within the nurse–patient relationship, both describe the use of emotional distancing and non-verbal cues that indicate dislike of an individual and which lead to a person feeling emotionally excluded.

Kelly and May (1982) argue that unless nurses are supported in exploring and challenging the social pressures to stereotype and exhibit prejudice, then their inability to provide non-judgemental care will continue. Rather than continuing to shame and berate practitioners for their apparent inadequacies, these authors propose the introduction of mechanisms whereby practitioners can discuss their beliefs and reflect on how these beliefs and values may affect care delivery.

While the concepts of reflection and supervision within clinical practice should not be seen as a panacea, their skilled and judicious use should enable nurses to become more self-aware (Critchley, 1987) and to reduce the stress associated with dependence upon maladaptive coping mechanisms such as denial, suppression and avoidance.

Sexual harassment and sexual abuse: distortions of gender and power

> 'The assumption that all social relations are gendered ... changes the nature of the debate from an exclusive focus on women to a focus on how gender shapes and is implicated in all kinds of social phenomena ...'
>
> (Acker, 1989, p.77)

Certain types of inappropriate behaviour in the healthcare context, and more specifically within the nurse–patient relationship, have their origins in the gendered abuse of power. The nursing press regularly contains reports of cases brought before the UKCC's professional conduct committee where different forms of abuse have taken place as a result of the misuse of power within the nurse–client relationship. Within our professional lives many of us will have witnessed what we may have considered inappropriate sexual relationships developing between nurses and current or ex patients/clients.

While illness and disability at any age can increase an individual's vulnerability, there are certain groups of clients who are more vulnerable to abuse than others. Later chapters in this book illustrate the professional nursing response to the sexual health needs of these more vulnerable groups, namely children, people with a learning disability, those with mental health problems and those who are physically frail.

In 1999, the UKCC published its first professional guidance for nurses on this subject *Practitioner–client relationships and the prevention of abuse.* A positive feature of this work is that there is overt acknowledgement of the strong emotional feelings that are often encountered when caring for an individual or family. There is also explicit support for the place of direct physical contact or touch as an integral facet of the therapeutic caring relationship.

However, a distinction is made between the natural or normal experience of such feelings and the consequences of acting upon them inappropriately within the professional relationship. In the UKCC guidance, practitioners are asked to consider the boundaries or limits of behaviour that serve to protect the best interests of not only the client but also the nurse. Nurse–patient relationships that focus more on meeting the practitioner's needs than those of the client are considered to represent '...an unacceptable abuse of power' (UKCC, 1999, p.5). The guidance also acknowledges the key contribution of nurse managers and employers in creating an organisational culture where abuse can be prevented through sound employment and supervision practices and makes recommendations for the early detection and management of abuse should it occur.

Another form of sexual abuse more prevalent in nursing is that of sexual harassment. Savage (1989) suggests that it is the combination of maternalism and sexual titillation within the public image of the nurse that contributes to the prevalence of sexual harassment within general nursing. Sexual harassment has probably always been part of nurses' lives and was a central consideration when Florence Nightingale established strict rules that governed nurses' behaviour as a means of protecting them against it (Bullough, 1990).

While sexual harassment is predominantly a problem faced by women in the workplace, this does not imply that men are not harassed. There is a dearth of research related to sexual harassment in nursing overall and currently no studies that address sexual harassment and men in nursing (Robbins *et al.*, 1997). The RCN's Employment Information and Research unit states that, in the absence of definitive figures, the exact extent of harassment and bullying experienced by nurses is unknown. However there is acknowledgement that both types of behaviour are significant issues for nurses and that there is a professional imperative to address the problem (RCN, 1997). The impact of negative professional stereotypes and the experience of harassment is at one and the same time both obvious/apparent and invisible within contemporary healthcare contexts and nursing practice.

One of the reasons for this apparent 'invisibility' is the problem of definition, with disagreement and discomfort surrounding what actually constitutes harassment. It would appear that innuendo and 'accidental' touching predominate as behaviours deemed to fall within this definition, although awareness of the perceived intent behind the behaviour is also considered pertinent (Horgan & Reeder, 1986). The RCN (1997, p.22) employment brief offers its own definition of harassment and outlines seven potential manifestations of sexual harassment within a model policy on harassment and bullying that can be modified by employers for local use.

In a review by Robbins, Bender and Finnis (1997) the authors expressed concern about the apparent reluctance among nurses to report incidents of harassment. This is particularly worrying when one considers the National Health Service to be the largest single employer of women in the UK.

An American survey by Grieco (1997) found that 76% of nurses who responded had experienced sexual harassment that ranged from inappropriate verbal comments to behaviour that could be defined as sexual assault. While patients were the most frequent source of this harassment (87%), medical (67%) and other colleagues (59%) also contributed to this destructive activity. Regrettably this study had a very low response rate (29% of sample) and so interpretation of these results is limited. As mentioned previously, qualitative research in Australia (Lawler, 1991) explored how nurses negotiate the boundaries of acceptable and unacceptable touch in the provision of intimate physical care. When patients transgressed these socially negotiated and implicit boundaries of acceptable behaviour the nursing response tended to be one of embarrassment and an attempt to use humour to laugh it off. Where the behaviour continued this was communicated to other nurses and avoidance was frequently used as a coping mechanism, with direct attention to the behaviour itself not generally encountered.

British research appears to concur with findings from the other countries previously mentioned, with rates of harassment ranging from 16% (Preston, 1990) to 97% (*Nursing Times* survey, 1993 cited in Finnis *et al.*) of respondents. Again, one of the major obstacles to interpretation of results is the influence of respondent bias where the non-response rate and their associated experiences are unknown. In a pilot study where 100% of nursing staff participated in interviews (Finnis *et al.*, 1993) 60% of the sample had experienced some form of sexual harassment from (male) patients, usually during the course of routine care such as assisting with personal hygiene. Again the nursing response was usually one of embarrassment and avoidance.

A more recent questionnaire survey (56% response rate) by Finnis and Robbins (1994) found that 66% of qualified nurses and 35% of student nurses had experienced sexual harassment, with patients as the most likely perpetrators, although for registered nurses there was an increasing tendency for male nursing staff or doctors to be responsible for this behaviour.

The body of literature pertaining to sexual harassment or impropriety of medical staff is also relatively scarce, although interest in the media portrayal of the doctor–patient relationship has increased substantially over recent years. A study of tabloid press coverage of professional misconduct cases brought before the General Medical Council (GMC) over a 17 month period revealed the media's increased interest in cases of alleged sexual misconduct compared to any other type of case (Bradby *et al.*, 1995). While other types of offence were more prevalent (23 out of 56 cases), it was the cases of sexual misconduct (15 out of 56 cases) which received most press attention, with 10 out of the 15 being reported compared to only 7 out of the remaining 41 cases where there were no allegations of sexual misconduct. In addition, the degree of coverage devoted to cases involving sex exceeded other misconduct case reporting.

What was more interesting than the rate of reporting, however, was the portrayal of male general practitioners as '...educated professionals who had succumbed to their "natural" sex urges while treating "busty blonde" female patients' (Bradby *et al.*, 1995, p.470). The authors of this study expressed concern that the tabloid press appeared to favour the promotion of a traditional gender ideology. The type of sexual motivation and behaviour that was acceptable for men and women remained narrowly defined and was frequently used to justify an abuse of professional power (Bradby *et al.*, 1995).

A larger body of research related to sexual abuse and harassment exists within the field of learning disability nursing, where the management of inappropriate or difficult sexual behaviour appears to receive more consistent professional attention as a legitimate aspect of client care and social education. However, a study by Thompson *et al.* (1997) reinforces findings from general nursing whereby female staff are forced to make individual responses to protect themselves from abuse due to the reluctance of learning disability services to identify '... the behaviour of men with learning difficulties as a concern for the whole agency and taking appropriate collective action' (p.574).

While these authors to do not disregard the men's disadvantage in their personal and sexual lives, they advocate the need for the sexual harassment and abuse of staff to be made visible and to be taken seriously given the inequalities experienced within the gendered hierarchies of service provision. Too often the strategies employed in resolving or reducing such negative behaviour are focused on the individual, thus ignoring the social and organisational context for the sexual harassment of nurses.

The positive and negative consequences of gender roles in society are brought into sharp relief within the microcosm of the hospital where traditional gender divisions of labour and the power base of a predominantly patriarchal society are prevalent and manifest in the 'doctor–patient–nurse' game that mirrors the traditional Victorian family structure (Katzman & Roberts, 1988).

Feminist writers such as Tong (1992) have suggested that such behaviour is a manifestation of abuse of power within a patriarchal system characterised by the use of dominance, hierarchy and competition to oppress women by virtue of their sexuality and gender. Robbins *et al.* (1997) conclude that for sexual harassment to succeed, certain conditions need to be fulfilled, namely collusion by the organisation to lack of recognition and/or inaction and a 'conspiracy of silence with the victim'. Until recently the healthcare system and professional nursing organisations have inadvertently supported these conditions through the maintenance of organisational cultures that fail to encourage true multi-professional integration, power sharing and team working or to recognise the complexity and sensitivity inherent in much of professional nursing activity.

As a result nurses and patients continue to be placed at risk within the context of both sexual health provision and nursing care delivery, with nurses unwilling to report such incidents due to embarrassment, guilt or rationalisation that the patient 'couldn't help it'. The nurse's silence can then be misinterpreted by both the perpetrator and by nurse managers as colluding with or even encouraging such behaviour and so cycles of harassment continue (Robbins *et al.*, 1997), exacerbated by the fact that the nurse may be unwilling or unable to remove herself from this situation because of a duty of care to the patient/client. Many nurses appear to be unaware that sexual harassment is one of the circumstances under which a registered practitioner can consider the withdrawal of 'duty to care' as a legitimate professional response where there is a need for self-protection (UKCC, 1996).

It remains important to note that sexual harassment takes place within a wider social context where there is still a tendency to place 'responsibility' for such incidents on the woman who is either ridiculed for being a 'humourless feminist' who could not take a joke or a 'sexual siren' who 'led the poor man on'. Such stereotypes demean not only the man and woman in this interaction but also the nature and intent of professional nursing action. It is imperative that at an organisational level, specific policies and training approaches are developed that both raise awareness of this problem and attend to the identification, reporting and management of sexual abuse and harassment. Such policies should include support of nurses who have experienced harassment. In this way, as with other forms of oppressive and discriminatory behaviour, sexual abuse and harassment will not be tolerated within the practitioner–client relationship or the workplace.

Conclusions

This chapter has attempted to place the individual practitioner's response to sexuality issues within its wider professional context, one that acknowledges both the overt and covert influences upon nursing knowledge and action within this domain of care. It has become increasingly difficult to create the ideal circumstances for more complex care needs to be met due to competing demands on the nursing role. Yet at no time has the actual and potential contribution of nursing been more readily acknowledged both within the profession and at governmental level (DoH, 1999).

In raising awareness of sexual issues in health care, nurses remain in a prime position to identify need, to provide information, support and to act in a liaison capacity for specialist psychosexual services where relevant. While clinical supervision is not a panacea, its provision can enhance opportunities for the development and maintenance of effective professional practice in order to meet the ever changing sexual health needs of clients we meet within both health and illness contexts. However, if individual practitioners are to fully realise their potential there must also be an appropriate organisational culture that provides the managerial support and development for staff who work with the complex and challenging issue of human sexuality. Such an organisational culture must also be capable of promoting non-prejudicial practice and creating zero tolerance of abuse and harassment for clients, their partners and healthcare professionals alike.

References

Aber, C.S. & Hawkins, J.W. (1992) Portrayal of nurses in advertisements in medical and nursing journals. IMAGE: *Journal of Nursing Scholarship*, **24**, 4, 289–93.

Acker, J. (1989) Making gender visible. Cited in C. Davies (1995) *Gender and the Professional Predicament in Nursing*. Open University Press, Buckingham.

Bancroft, J. (1989) *Human Sexuality and its Problems* (second edition, Chapter 6: Homosexuality). Churchill Livingstone, Edinburgh.

Bernhard, L.A. & Dan, A.J. (1986) Redefining sexuality from women's own experiences. *Nursing Clinics of North America*, **21**, 1, 125–36.

Bradby, H., Gabe, J. & Bury, M. (1995) 'Sexy docs' and 'busty blondes': press coverage of professional misconduct cases brought before the General Medical Council. *Sociology of Health & Illness*, **17**, 4, 458–76.

Bullough, V.L. (1990) Nightingale, nursing and harassment. *Journal of Nursing Scholarship*, **22**, 1, 4–7.

Bullough, V.L. & Seidl, A. (1987) Attitudes on sexuality in nursing texts today and yesterday. *Holistic Nursing Practice*, **1**, 4, 84–92.

Critchley, D.L. (1987) Clinical supervision as a learning tool for the therapist in milieu settings. *Journal of Psychosocial Nursing and Mental Health Services*, **25**, 8, 18–22.

Davies, C. (1995) *Gender and the Professional Predicament in Nursing*. Open University Press, Buckingham.

DoH (1999) *Making a Difference: Strengthening the nursing, midwifery and health visiting contribution to health and healthcare*. Department of Health, London.

Douglas, C.J. (1985) Homophobia amongst physicians and nurses; an empirical study. *Hospital and Community Psychiatry*, **36**, 1309–11.

Evans, J. (1997) Men in nursing: issues of gender segregation and hidden advantage. *Journal of Advanced Nursing*, **26**, 226–31.

Fagin, C. & Diers, D. (1984) Nursing as metaphor. *International Nursing Review*, **31**, 16–17.

Fiedler, L.A. (1988) Images of the nurse in fiction and popular culture. In: A. Hudson Jones (ed.) *Images of Nursing: Perspectives from History, Art and Literature*. University of Pennsylvania Press, Philadelphia.

Finnis, S.J. & Robbins, I. (1994) Sexual harassment of nurses: An occupational hazard. *Journal of Clinical Nursing*, **3**, 87–95.

Finnis, S.J., Robbins, I. & Bender, M.P. (1993) A pilot study of the prevalence and psychological sequelae of sexual harassment of nursing staff. *Journal of Clinical Nursing*, **3**, 23–7.

Goffman, E. (1968) *Stigma: Notes on the management of a spoiled identity.* Prentice-Hall, Englewood Cliffs, NJ.

Grieco, A. (1987) Scope and nature of sexual harassment in nursing. *Journal of Sex Research*, **23**, 2, 261–6.

Hacker, S.S. (1984) Students' questions about sexuality: Implications for nurse educators. *Nurse Educator*, Winter, 28–31.

Hayter, M. (1996) Is non-judgemental care possible in the context of nurses' attitudes to patients' sexuality? *Journal of Advanced Nursing*, **24**, 662–6.

Hite, S. (1976) *The Hite Report.* Dell, New York.

Horgan, D.D. & Reeder, G. (1986) Sexual harassment in nursing, *AAOHN Journal*, **34**, 2, 83–6.

Hunter, K.M. (1988) Nurses: the satiric image and the translocated ideal. In: A. Hudson Jones (ed.). *Images of Nursing: Perspectives from History, Art and Literature.* University of Pennsylvania Press, Philadelphia.

Johnson, M. & Webb, C. (1995) Rediscovering the unpopular patient: the concept of social judgement. *Journal of Advanced Nursing*, **21**, 1112–17.

Kalisch, P.A. & Kalisch, B.J. (1982a) Nurses on prime-time television. *American Journal of Nursing*, **82**, 2, 265–70.

Kalisch, P.A. & Kalisch, B.J. (1982b) The image of the nurse in motion pictures. *American Journal of Nursing*, **82**, 4, 605–11.

Kalisch, P.A. & Kalisch, B.J. (1982c) The image of nurses in novels. *American Journal of Nursing*, **82**, 8, 1220–24.

Kalisch, P.A. & Kalisch, B.J. (1986) A comparative analysis of nurse and physician characters in the entertainment media. *Journal of Advanced Nursing*, **11**, 179–95.

Katzman, E.M. & Roberts, J.I. (1988) Nurse–physician conflicts as barriers to the enactment of nursing roles. *Western Journal of Nursing Research*, **10**, 5, 576–90.

Kautz, D.D., Dickey, C.A. & Stevens, M.N. (1990) Using research to identify why nurses do not meet established sexuality nursing care standards. *Journal of Nursing Quality Assurance*, **4**, 3, 67–9.

Kelly, M.P. & May, D. (1982) Good and bad patients: a review of the literature and a theoretical critique. *Journal of Advanced Nursing*, **7**, 147–56.

Kinsey, A.C., Pomeray, W.B., Martin, C.E. & Gephard, P.H. (1953) *Sexual Behavior in the Human Female.* W.B. Saunders, Philadelphia.

Lawler, J. (1991) *Behind the Screens: Nursing, Somology and the Problem of the Body.* Churchill Livingstone, Edinburgh.

Lewis, S. & Bor, R. (1994) Nurses' knowledge of and attitudes towards sexuality and the relationship of these with nursing practice. *Journal of Advanced Nursing*, **20**, 2, 251–9.

Masters, W.H. & Johnson, V.E. (1966) *Human Sexual Response*. Little Brown & Co, Boston.

Porter, S. (1992) Women in a women's job: the gendered experience of nurses. *Sociology of Health and Illness*, **14**, 4, 510–27.

Preston, A. (1990) Sexual Harassment Survey. *Nursing Standard*, **5**, 1, 62–3.

Pryce, A. (1991) Sexuality and the patient. *Nursing*, **4**, 44, 15–16.

Robbins, I., Bender, M.P. & Finnis, S.J. (1997) Sexual harassment in nursing. *Journal of Advanced Nursing*, **25**, 163–9.

Royal College of Nursing (1997) *Employment Brief 13/97: Harassment and Bullying at Work*. RCN Employment Information and Research Unit, London.

Savage, J. (1989) Sexuality: An univited guest. *Nursing Times*, **85**, 5, 25–8.

Sundeen, S.J., Stuart, G.W., Rantan, E.A.D. & Cohen S.A. (1989) *Nurse–Client Interaction: Implementing the Nursing Process* (fifth edition). C.V. Mosby, St Louis.

Thompson, D., Clare, I. & Brown, H. (1997) Not such an 'ordinary' relationship: the role of women support staff in relation to men with learning disabilities who have difficult sexual behaviour. *Disability and Society*, **12**, 4, 573–92.

Tong, R. (1992) *Feminist Thought*. Routledge, London.

United Kingdom Central Council (UKCC) for Nursing, Midwifery and Health Visiting (1992) *Code of Professional Conduct* (third edition). UKCC, London.

United Kingdom Central Council (UKCC) for Nursing, Midwifery and Health Visiting (1996) *Guidelines for Professional Practice*. UKCC, London.

United Kingdom Central Council (UKCC) for Nursing, Midwifery and Health Visiting (1999) *Practitioner–client relationships and the Prevention of Abuse*. UKCC, London.

Webb, C.A. (1988) A study of nurses' knowledge and attitudes about sexuality in health care. *International Journal of Nursing Studies*, **25**, 3, 235–44.

White, I.D. (1994) *Nurses' social construction of sexuality within a cancer care context: an exploratory case study*. Unpublished MSc Nursing thesis, City University, London.

5. Nurses, the Body and Body Work

Hazel Heath with Brendan McCormack

Whenever nurses work with patients they engage in body work of some kind. Both nurse and patient are living within, and communicating through, the medium of their bodies. Body work is central to nursing practice in that, to varying degrees according to individual need, nurses are concerned with the care and functioning of other people's bodies. Body work is complex and continually challenging for both patients and nurses. Nurses must learn to renegotiate social norms within their relationships with patients in order to care for their bodies while at the same time assisting them through their experiences of bodily changes during illness and towards death.

The human body is biological, comprising highly complex interrelated physiological systems, yet biological explanations alone are insufficient to explain the experience of living in a body. We live in our bodies, yet are more than our bodies. The body is the medium through which we experience our lives and is also the showcase of our inner being. It is central to our perception of self and therefore to the construction of our identities. The bodies of others are similarly showcases on which we may make judgements; are central in the construction of their identities and are also the medium through which we engage in our relationships with them.

This chapter highlights why body work is an issue in nursing practice, together with some of the key challenges for nurses. It discusses how body work can become sexualised. It explores a range of perspectives on how the body has been viewed in literature and, specifically, the kinds of changes that people with illness or disability can experience.

Body work: challenges in nursing

Patients' bodies and bodily functions are central in nursing, even when there is no direct physical contact between the patient and nurse. Nurses care for people's bodies in a range of ways which aim to minimise the effects of illness and disability and to maximise health and independence. The degree and type of direct bodily care will vary according to individual need but will likely increase as a person's health deteriorates or they become increasingly dependent on others. Body work in nursing can be highly challenging for a variety of reasons.

Person-centred and holistic care

Patients' bodies are subject to the attention of a wide range of healthcare professionals but most focus on a particular aspect of bodily function. For example, a general physician will review the functioning of bodily cells and systems; a cardiologist will focus on cardiovascular functioning; radiographers take X-rays; phlebotomists take blood, etc. Focusing on one aspects of bodily function can allow professionals to remain distanced from the patient as an individual person and the body can become a 'thing' – a biologically functioning object of study.

Such distancing is not appropriate for nurses. They must interact with the patient at times when the body and its functioning are a central concern; through illness and towards death. In order to offer person-centred and holistic care, nurses must engage with the living experience of each patient in his or her body and how bodily changes affect that lived experience. In this way it can be more difficult for nurses to view the body as a 'thing' or object detached from the patient's individual being.

One example of nursing's challenges in engaging closely with patients both as persons and as bodies is when patients die. From her research on how nurses work with bodies, Lawler concluded that a great deal of discomfort, even fearfulness and cultural superstition, attends dealing with dead bodies. This can be increased by the technical advances that have blurred divisions between life and death. Patients may be 'clinically dead' but their bodily functioning is maintained by technological and care support. In this situation the person is warm and treated as if he/she is still alive but does the nurse consider the personality as dead?

Perceptions of body work

In traditional hierarchies of nursing work technical tasks, and particularly those which emulate the work of doctors, have been highly valued. Body work has traditionally been viewed as menial and delegated to assistants. Body work is also commonly perceived as essentially a female role in that it encompasses activities that mothers undertake for their children (such as washing, feeding, toileting). This can influence how male nurses are perceived, and brings additional challenges for their practice.

Perception of body work as menial also affects how various client groups are perceived. Those requiring more body care have traditionally been perceived negatively. As Adams and Keady (2001) describe: 'the association with ... leakage of fluids such as urine and faeces from the body often leads to the marginalisation of dementia care nursing and its labelling as "dirty work".'

Body work is perceived negatively by non-nurses and even by patients who have experienced nursing at first hand. For example, following hospitalisation, patients might say:

> ' "nurses are wonderful, worth a lot more money" ... they would not go home and say "the nurses are really wonderful, they took really good care of my bowel" ... they wouldn't talk about it. They will talk about "my operation", "my doctor" but they won't talk so much about the pan and having the enema and how the nurse did the enema or "washed me" or all that sort of thing ... [It is] soon forgotten and locked away ... they go back into a situation where those things aren't talked about ... so I think people who have never been hospitalised do not know what nurses do, and even those who have been hospitalised won't tell them'.
>
> (Lawler, 1991, pp.224–5)

Nakedness and bodily touch

Body care results in patients' bodies being exposed in ways which normally only occur in highly private situations and nurses often need to touch patients' bodies in areas which are usually only touched by others in intimate relationships. In these ways everyday nursing work violates social norms and conventions and this can be challenging for both patients and nurses.

Nurses must construct a context and method of working in which it becomes permissible, and as comfortable as possible for all parties, for them to undress people, see their naked bodies and even genitalia, and touch these where necessary. Nurses deal with body work in a range of ways such as creating a 'clinical' environment;

using a 'professional' approach; adopting biomedical (non-every-day) language. These all help to play down the 'personal' elements within a situation and to minimise any sexual connotations, but there are challenges in this.

Language

Although biomedical terminology is commonly used, nurse and patient language needs to be adapted to individual interactions. Nurses should attempt to use terms which the other person can readily understand. This can present a range of challenges, as nurses in Lawler's (1991) interviews explained, including embarrassment or lack of confidence, lack of adequate education and the individual backgrounds of the nurse and/or the patient. One remarked:

> 'It's definitely class related. Joe Bloggs off the river bank is easy to talk to. They shit, they fart, they piss. You can communicate. It's the people with a middle-class presentation you don't have the vocabulary to match.'
>
> (Lawler, 1991, p.132)

Unpleasant work

Dealing with people's bodies, bodily functions, bodily fluids, particularly when they are ill or dying, can be unpleasant and nurses routinely deal with sights, smells and activities which would be repugnant to many (Lawler, 1991, p.48). Nurses must learn to cope with such situations physically and psychologically and, in addition, must take precautions to protect themselves, for example from exposure to potentially contaminated body fluids. Crucially, they must do all of this in a manner which does not treat the body as an object and thus does not 'objectify' or 'disembody' the patient but instead acknowledges his or her embodied experience.

Sexualisation of body work

Nursing as an occupation is commonly ascribed attributes and connotations of sexuality and this potentially imbues nurse–patient encounters with sexual meaning. Engaging through and with the bodies of others takes place on a range of levels but is inherently sexualised (see Chapter 4 for a full discussion). Lawler (1991, p.107) believes that

> 'The body and sexuality are indivisible, the body is a sexualised construct which impacts on social life and vice versa, and it

influences the way people interact with each other. This is clearly illustrated in studies about which areas of other people's bodies it is socially permissible to touch'.

In addition, nurses often work with people at their most vulnerable. They touch their bodies in a kindly, caring and soothing way. They try to promote comfort, relaxation and wellbeing. Bodily touch, particularly of this type, stimulates the senses and is therefore, of essence, sensual. Within a non-healthcare context, such contact could be construed as a sexual invitation (Lawler, 1991, p.212).

Because of this sexuality and body work are to some extent inseparable, but some areas of the body are particularly sexualised, such as genitalia. The issue is obviously distinct between the genders. There is little research on how male nurses feel about working with female genitalia. Lawler (1991, p.195) suggests that, compared with female sexuality and femininity, male sexuality and masculinity are more genital and physical constructs but admits that her research is strongly focused on the perceptions of female nurses to the detriment of male nurse perspectives.

For female nurses, washing a penis can be difficult or embarrassing.

> 'You never wash it . . . you wash down as far as it and you come as far as it, and then you give them the soapy washer [and if they weren't able to wash it] you washed it as quickly as you could! And talked! . . . anything that came into your head (laughter).'
> (Lawler, 1991, p.200)

Female nurses also experience embarrassment and lack of confidence in dealing with erections, although distinction is made between whether these are perceived to be intentional or accidental.

The few male nurses in Lawler's research did not identify either male or female sexual behaviour as a problem for them, except in situations where they felt this was deliberate. Both male and female nurses did not tolerate deliberate exposure. One male nurse in Lawler's (1991, p.202) research, managed the situation of an accidental erection by pretending it wasn't there: 'and by the time the erection is at full mast I've nearly finished and you can roll them over and [wash] their backs ... I mean it must be fairly embarrassing'.

Body work with some patients is deemed to be less imbued with sexual meaning. For very ill people the priority of the life or death situation can be perceived as placing less threat of a sexualised incident (see Chapter 13), and also in very old people, where sex is usually perceived to be less relevant (see Chapter 9).

Nursing literature on body work

Although literature from a range of disciplines has explored the body, no single perspective has yet fully accommodated it theoretically. In addition, literature in the field of health care tends towards reductionism, with each discipline having its distinct focus. Nursing has generated little literature on the body, Lawler's work (1991, 1997) being the notable exception. Nursing knowledge of the body is not generally valued. Being practical knowledge, knowledge embedded in practice, it is regarded as emotional rather than rational knowledge and not relying heavily on intellect. It is also dependent on situations and the persons involved.

Perspectives on the body

Philosophical perspectives

The body has been discussed extensively in philosophical writings but the philosophical literature reflects a dominant interest in mind as opposed to body. Where the body has been discussed, it is against a background of human experience.

Descartes (1986, p.159) recognised the metaphysical difficulty of both having, and being a body. To him is attributed the origin of the concept of a distinction between mind and body – Cartesian dualism.

Harré (1986, p.190) argued that a person simultaneously 'owns' a body, experiences it and exists in it. The body as an object must be integrated with the body as experience. Sartre (circa 1960, p.344) wrote about the self as mediated by the interpersonal and intrapersonal aspects of embodiment. To Sartre, the body is both a being for itself, an object perceived as a personal sense of embodiment, and a being for others in that it functions as both an instrument of, and for, social interaction with others. For Sartre, personhood and embodiment require each other.

Merleau-Ponty (1962, p.82) emphasised the need to locate the body in context, particularly in time and space, and he argues that the centrality of the body in the development of identity and interpersonal being is integral to human existence. The body also has a private notion of who we are and how we interact with each other. For humans therefore the qualities of *having* and *being* a body are both material and non-material and, while the body expresses our existence, it cannot be reduced to experience (Merleau-Ponty, 1962, p.166).

Historical and symbolic perspectives

The human body has historically been a rich and potent symbol, both secular and sacred, throughout history. Greek and Roman sculptures bear witness to the admiration of the body in ancient cultures. Images in modern history and contemporary culture similarly depict current societal views on the 'ideal body' or 'the body beautiful'. At any point in history, and within each social context, there is widespread understanding of the desirable attributes of the human body but this fluctuates from century to century and decade to decade.

Body rituals (such as circumcision, baptism, body markings or cutting) are also used in religious and cultural contexts to mark rites of passage, status, or the inclusion of an individual into the corpus of that society. The body has been represented as being sacred (for example when the body and blood of Christ are symbolically shared during Holy Communion) or profane, dangerous and to be avoided (for example taboos or rituals surrounding bodily fluids, particularly menstrual blood and semen).

Rituals surrounding death of the body also illustrate a range of perspectives. A body may be buried intact if the person, as a body, is no longer viewed as having a sustainable existence. Alternatively, bodies may be burned if the prevailing view is that their usefulness has ended and the essence, or soul, of what was the person has gone elsewhere.

Sociological perspectives

We experience our bodies within a social context. Prevailing social and cultural norms determine what, in terms of bodies, is viewed as normal, desirable, acceptable or unacceptable. Social or cultural norms and roles also determine what we do with our bodies, how they are presented, what is exposed and what remains covered, how we use our bodies and how we control bodily functions. Social and cultural rules also determine boundaries in our relationships with others, for example what, where, how and when it is socially acceptable to touch other people. These rules are also determined by context or subculture, for example the touching of another's genitals may be permissible for a doctor or professional sex worker but would be differently construed outside the professional context.

Society also influences our attitudes towards our own bodies and the concept of body image has been theorised from a range of perspectives. Our body image is shaped not just by our perception of our body's appearance, but how this perception is mediated by our social and cultural context. This image will impact upon our sense of self, our confidence and social relationships and how we experience our bodies in everyday life.

In contemporary western society there is considerable emphasis on body shape, style and fashion. Competitive individuals select the most advantageous strategies for the presentation of themselves and their bodies. These usually include manipulation of hairstyle and clothing but plastic surgery, for both women and men, is now increasingly selected as a means of adjusting body shape to present a particular identity.

People who fall outside society's preferred bodily characteristics can experience stigmatisation, particularly people who are disfigured or disabled. For example, Williams and Barlow (1998) discuss how men and women with arthritis feared their altered bodies might undermine how people felt about them and had made particular efforts to bring their perceived body image more in line with ideal images. Fairhurst (1998) described how, in contemporary society, older people felt a tension between being 'appropriately old' and adjusting their appearance with an attendant risk of being thought of as 'mutton dressed as lamb'.

Gender

Any culture determines what are 'natural' attributes for males and females in terms of body appearance, presentation and functioning, but these determinations extend beyond biological differences to prescribed roles and ways of behaving. Seymour (1989, p.16) suggests that the female monopoly on reproduction has associated women with the essentially 'private' and domestic domain of child rearing and family life. The male's distance from the pragmatics of reproduction aligns him in the more 'public' domain of the real world. Seymour highlights that, although there are obvious biological and bodily differences between men and women, gender identity is further emphasised by socialisation into specific gender roles and attributes. Many current debates highlight these issues. For example, are debates about whether women soldiers should fight in frontline battle based on biological/bodily differences or generally prescribed gender attributes and roles? A debate has been raised as to whether two genders are sufficient to encompass the range of ways in which individuals wish to express themselves. Some individuals wish to be be labelled as neither male nor female and the term 'intergender' has been suggested.

Embodiment

Embodiment is a concept discussed in literature from a range of perspectives. The literature highlights that we *have* bodies, but we *are* bodies. The consciousness of human beings is invariably embedded within the body. Berger and Luckman (1967, p.68) state that 'our embodiment is essential for our social being. A person experiences him or herself as an entity not identical with the body, but one that has a body at his or her disposal'. Turner (1984, p.233) describes:

> 'I can touch, feel, smell and see my body, but I need my body in order to carry out these activities of touching, feeling, smelling and seeing. I possess my body in a much more thorough and immediate sense than I could ever possess other objects. Yet also I possess my body in this thoroughgoing sense, the very intimacy of possession is the source of my destruction, since the death of my body is also my death.'

Leder (1992, p.25) suggests that

> 'we cannot understand the meaning and form of objects without reference to bodily powers through which we engage them – our senses, motility, language, desires. The lived body is not just one thing in the world but a way in which the world comes to be'.

Most of the time we are unaware of our bodies during normal function but at other times we become more aware. This naturally occurs at particular times of life, for example during adolescence or ageing, when our bodies change in the way in which they look and function.

Social and cultural concepts of bodily health

Health is multidimensional and bodily functioning is a key element of this. How an individual perceives and feels his or her body is fundamental to self-perception and identity but societal and cultural perceptions also influence how bodies, bodily functioning and health/illness are perceived. Seymour (1989) suggests that a healthy body is seen as being controlled, in order and in balance with nature. Practices of body regulation such as hygiene, exercise, sleep and sexual continence are designed in order to maintain healthy bodies but are as political as they are functional. In contemporary society, people who seek to help themselves by engaging in such activities gain social approval, not because they are social conformists, but rather, Seymour suggests, because healthy bodies are seen as normal and unthreatening to the status quo.

> 'Health is normal. Health is life in balance with nature. Health is order. Ill health is abnormal, a body out of balance with nature, in disarray and disorder. Health is the resolution of the tension between bodily control and social control: it results from the regulation of the anarchy of the body by the civilising forces of society.'
>
> (Seymour, 1989, p.28)

This idea is taken further by Turner (1984) who suggests that social order can be directly related to issues of body regulation; that social order depends on the resolution of the perpetual tension between desire and discipline, between anarchy and order, between the body and society. According to Turner, illness and disease can be seen as a result of the body's ability or refusal to conform to society's prescriptions. If health is normality, ill health is deviancy – the unhealthy person is a deviant.

Societal and cultural contexts not only influence and give meaning to perceptions of health and illness but also to bodily changes and symptoms. Zola (1973, p.680) argues that, since there are no inherent physiological differences between members of different social classes or ethnic groups, variations in ideas about health and illness are culturally derived. Zola uses the example of research which suggests that western women feel more pain during childbirth than women in Papua New Guinea and questions whether the former group could be imagining their pain or the latter are especially stoical.

Prevailing social and cultural norms control physiological functioning in many areas of life such as the selection, preparation and eating of food. This in turn regulates the body's desire to eat, the elimination of bodily waste and practices for child rearing (e.g. feeding and toilet training). Social/cultural norms change over time, even within single cultures, as ideas change, for example about the desirability of eating saturated fats.

Internal bodily control

The importance of bodily control is a constant theme in the literature and the ability to control one's body can be critical in maintaining our social status, yet the interior of the body is not easy to control and how our internal organs behave is usually inaccessible to us. Seymour (1989, p.11) describes the interior of the body as 'a context for anarchy', particularly as 'our well tended bodies may at any time betray our years of faithful love and care' when our internal organs turn against us. Common within the literature on ageing are expressions of the experience of, or the fear of, losing the capacity to undertake activities which one has taken for granted at a younger age. The ultimate loss of such capacities is loss of independence in managing one's own body and subsequent dependence on others to do so. Featherstone and Hepworth (1991, p.376) observe that

> 'loss of bodily control carries similar penalties of stigmatisation and ultimately physical exclusion ... degrees of loss impair the capacity to be counted as a competent adult. Indeed, the failure of bodily controls can lead to a more general loss of self image; to be ascribed the status of a competent adult person depends upon the capacity to control urine and faeces'.

Loss of body control does not only arise in illness. Breastfeeding mothers have described their bodies as having 'minds of their own' when their breasts involuntarily leaked milk. Britton (1998) taped focus group interviews with 30 post-natal women aged 20–39 from a variety of backgrounds in terms of class, religion and ethnicity. These mothers described the feeling of their bodies letting them down and embarrassing them but also of their bodies having a separate, dissociated identity in that they were unable to control them. The mothers then experienced a paradox between trying to control the leakage most of the time, yet trying to relax and allow the leakage while the baby was feeding.

Exercising control over one's body can also be used as a means of control in acts of 'social rebellion'. The obese body has come to signify a body out of control. By means of hunger strikes and anorexia nervosa the body asserts its supremacy over society. Bulimia represents a personal expression of the tension between desire and the social criteria of appropriate body size and shape, especially for women (Seymour, 1989, p.18).

Control over the internal body is viewed as the province of doctors in that they know how to identify changes and symptoms and how to investigate and treat these. There is also control in this scenario in that a body may not reveal to the patient what is actually happening, and some doctors may choose whether or not to tell patients what they have found.

Illness and the meaning of illness

Illness changes how a person's body looks, feels and functions. Diseases carry social and cultural labels that reflect dominant societal views on what is acceptable. This is particularly so with sexually transmitted infections (see Chapters 3 and 12), but is also true of eating disorders such as anorexia or bulimia nervosa where societal expectations of appearance may conflict with an individual's self-perception (Turner, 1984, p.112).

Seymour (1989, p.29) suggests that the states of body that come to be seen as normal are those that conform to the ideas of a dominant group in society. A body out of order indicates that society is out of order. If such a deviation cannot be managed, then the unhealthy body (e.g. obese, disfigured or disabled people) will have to be marginalised – pushed to the periphery of society, not accounted for, out of sight – lest it should distract others from devotion of the dominant ideology, which is health and normalcy.

A diagnosis confirms physiological changes but also creates a framework of assumptions and expectations around the individual diagnosis. Different body parts may have different meanings for individuals, both real and symbolic, for example the heart. Seymour (1989) suggests that the heart is the essential organ for life but that it is shrouded in symbolism; for example as the seat of emotions. This can affect how a person adjusts to a heart attack, open heart surgery or heart transplant. Reconstructing one's identity with someone else's heart could be a challenging process. The breast, like the heart, is embedded in symbolism and social meaning. To be a woman is to have breasts. After mastectomy the task of reconstitution of self as a woman, as a sexual being and as a mother, can be formidable in the face of the strong social attitudes associated with this organ.

Transitions in illness

We usually take our bodies for granted and tend to notice them only when there is an alteration in how they feel or function. When illness occurs we become aware that our bodies are different and we may not be able to control them as previously. This changes our feelings towards our bodies and our relationships with them. This in turn affects our self-identity, how we relate to others and, consequently, our relationships with them. In situations of severe illness or trauma, when we need care or even hospitalisation, our identity changes from that of 'person' to 'patient'.

Seymour (1989, p.72) describes the experiences of transition following sudden limb paralysis. The initial loss of functioning of parts of the physical body infringe a person's self-understanding as the paralysis has become, in effect, separated from the identity of the paralysed person. The reality of the physical loss is unequivocal but the conceptual understanding of that reality is not so clear. The physical body is no longer appropriate to the concept of self, and readjustment to the new physical reality is usually a long and difficult process.

The various pieces of equipment necessary in the early days of paralysis, such as respirators, nasogastric tubes and urinary catheters, collude to confirm that the individual's identity is now that of a paralysed patient. Former components of an individual's sense of self – of being a father, a businessman etc. become deconstituted. The new self with which the person is confronted is that of paraplegic or quadriplegic, but for someone to identify with this is very challenging.

A person's identity is also built into relationships, e.g. a hospitalised husband to his wife. This too is changed in that, during the early stages of being in hospital the wife is not with him in their home, she becomes a visitor to the hospital. They are no longer able to interact or be intimate, as previously; she may appear to be siding with hospital staff in 'managing' him and may even become his full-time carer.

Seymour (1989, p.74) suggests that, in such a situation, a person's identity must, in time, be deconstituted as the new physical condition becomes more familiar. Gradually the previously taken for granted assumptions about the everyday world can be challenged and the person's former interests and concerns confronted. Some may prove to be inappropriate in the current situation and are negated; others are incorporated into the new reality. Then, through a gradual process of identity deconstruction and reconstruction, a new personal and social reality can be developed and the individual can develop a sense of what life might be like in the future. This process can take a long time.

Loss of a body part, e.g. amputation, presents another vivid example of the separation of body and self-image. Although many logical medical explanations exist for phantom limb sensations, such sensations may, in part, relate to the lack of realignment of self-image with the new body state (Seymour, 1989).

Williams (1996) illustrates this process of identity deconstruction and reconstruction in chronic illness. When the illness first arises, the person is likely to have been previously in a state of 'embodiment', i.e. the body is taken for granted in everyday life. During relapses into disease, a sense of 'dys-embodiment' is experienced, i.e. the dysfunctional state becomes the embodied experience. There follows an oscillation between states of 'dys-embodiment' to 're-embodiment' during subsequent relapses and remissions of bodily symptoms. Williams (1996) suggests that these attempts to move from a dys-embodied state to a re-embodied state require a considerable amount of 'biographical work', or what Williams (1984) terms 'narrative reconstruction'.

In studying people who are dying, Glaser and Strauss (1965, p.79) note that, despite awareness in both staff and the patient that the patient is dying, there is a complex ambiguity for the patient. The experience of their dying as yet has no meaning for them. Each experience and meaning must be established anew in each new situation.

Caring for people and their bodies

When working with people whose bodies have undergone transitions through illness, disability, advanced ageing, or approaching death, there is a great deal that nurses and others can do to help. This section offers some ideas.

Maintaining personhood

Personhood is a concept developed by Kitwood (1993a, b) when working with people with dementia. In many physical illnesses the patient's physical body can change but the patient as a person is still intact. Dementia produces the reverse effect. Although people with dementia have an organic illness that totally changes their lives, their bodies tend not to look greatly different to how they did before they were ill. The person, however, can appear to be lost. This can be a terrifying experience for the person and those close to him or her. As Kitwood (1993a, p.16) describes 'not only are they losing such everyday faculties as memory, planning and judgement; they are losing the very basis for knowing the nature of their predicament, and ultimately for holding onto who they are'. Kitwood argues that, in this situation, there can be a tendency to manipulate the individual and thus turn the person into an object.

When someone's body is changing, whatever the cause, maintaining personhood and personal worth is of vital importance. Kitwood (1993b) describes personhood as involving unique subjectivity, needs, rights, place in the human group and value for no instrumental purpose but simply as an end. For personal worth we must feel wanted, be able to make choices and to have an effect on the world in which we live.

The manifestations of diseases are not solely a matter of what changes have taken place in the physical body. For example Kitwood (1993b) emphasises that a person's dementia is not merely a matter of what has happened in their brains and neurological systems. It is also influenced by a combination of body-related factors, i.e. health (acute and chronic physical or mental health) and the neurological impairment, but also manifests other factors such as personality (personal resources – both positive and negative), biographical experience and the social psychology of what is happening in people's ordinary lives. Kitwood highlights the evidence that social events cause biochemical changes in the body (for example the effects of anxiety on physical state).

In order to help maintain personhood, nurses and others working with patients must 'discover the person, not the disease' (Kitwood, 1993b, p.16). This can involve the removal of traditional barriers between 'them' (the patients) and 'us' (the professionals) and based on what Kitwood describes as the 'painful truth that we and they belong to one humanity. All of us are damaged or deficient in some way. All of us have feelings, intentions and actions with meaning'. Drawing closer can be a profound and creative experience. 'As we discover the person ... we also discover something of ourselves, for what we ultimately have to offer is not technical expertise but our power to feel, to give, to stand in the shoes of another, through our imagination' (Kitwood, 1993b, p.17).

Support through transition

As people experience illness or other bodily change, they need to be able to integrate new and different ways of using their bodies and living within them. People may pass through periods of feeling dysembodied (as if their bodies do not belong to them) and then reembodied as new elements of understanding are incorporated. Each person's path through the process is different and he/she may need privacy and solitude, to talk at length, or to try out new experiences. New understandings can take a long time to integrate and it is important for healthcare workers to take their lead from the individual.

Body image

Body image is fundamental in adjusting to bodily changes. Various models have been offered. Price's model of body image care

(1990a, b) is conjectural but can be helpful. Price suggests that three major aspects feed an individual's body image:

- *body reality* is the body 'warts and all' (e.g. having undergone changes through illness, disability or treatment)
- *body ideal* is how we visualise our bodies should look and perform
- *body presentation* is how the body is presented to the outside world

Dissonance between body reality and body ideal can result in altered body image but the detrimental effects can, to some extent, be balanced by body presentation. Nurses can help considerably in this respect.

Body image is dynamic and constantly changing as perceptions are influenced by those around us and the feelings and experience of one's body. Pain and discomfort can considerably hinder a person's adjustment to changed body states and nurses can help in promoting comfort. There is now a great deal of nursing literature on how to minimise pain. White (1995, p.555) recommends establishing a relationship of mutual trust; using different types of pain-relief measures; providing pain relief before pain becomes severe; considering the patient's ability or willingness to participate in pain relief measures; choosing pain relief measures on the basis of the patient's behaviour indicating the severity of pain; using measures that the patient believes are effective; keeping an open mind about possible sources of pain relief and, even if pain relief does not appear to be working, to keep trying, reassess the situation, and consider alternatives.

Valuing body work

Contrary to the traditional hierarchy which values 'technical' tasks and relegates body work to the menial, many nurses continue to value body work as an integral aspect of their practice and to make opportunities to undertake it in order that they can maintain a close relationship with patients and monitor health status. This can be particularly valuable in long-term care settings (Heath, 2002, in preparation).

Touch

Each person has a predisposition to touch based on his/her own culture and life experience. Whilst nurses should try to recognise the influence of these when using touch in practice, touch can be a powerful way of reassuring individuals that their bodies are still 'touchable' and, by implication that they are still lovable. Colton (1983) suggests that touch hunger is analogous to malnutrition in that it results from the lack of adequate nutrients for bodily survival. Touch stimulates chemical production in the brain, which feeds blood, muscles, tissues, nerve cells, organs, and other body structures. Without this stimulation, like nutrients in food, the individual could be deprived of sustenance and could starve. Touch as a therapeutic strategy can be particularly effective with people who feel stigmatised or rejected through disfigurement, disability or a lesion such as a fungating wound.

Touch is a fundamental and universal aspect of nursing (Fisher & Joseph, 1989). It may be instrumental (deliberate and initiated to perform an act such as a wash), or expressive (spontaneous and showing feelings such as an expression of comfort). Touch can be used as a skilled nursing intervention, and to decrease sensory deprivation (leMay & Redfern, 1989). It can calm and reassure, comfort and soothe, and help people to feel valued (Fisher & Joseph, 1989; Fraser & Ross-Kerr, 1993). Moore and Gilbert's research (1995) showed that older residents of a nursing home perceived greater affection and intimacy when nurses used comforting touch and that higher or lower levels of affection are communicated during nurse–patient encounters. Their research suggested that adults in general rely more on non-verbal cues and that visual and hearing loss may reduce an older person's ability to derive meaning from non-verbal behaviours such as a nod or a smile. They may depend more on what they can feel, rather than see and hear. At a time when their need for touch was the greatest, the older people had begun to think of themselves as untouchable.

Nurses are increasingly expanding their practice with the use of a range of complementary therapies which can help patients to relax, increase their awareness of their bodies and consequently adjust to changes more easily.

Body work practice

In the manner in which they conduct their day-to-day work with patients and their bodies, nurses can do a great deal to help people feel valued as individuals, however they are feeling about their own bodies. When touching bodies, adjusting body boundaries with the use of equipment, handling bodily fluids or monitoring bodily functions, nurses can show recognition of the patient as a person, and sensitivity to their feelings and experiences at that particular time. For example, Stutchfield (2000) observes that many patients who have undergone stoma surgery feel shame, stigma, rejection and social isolation. The stoma can even become the dominant aspect in a person's daily life. Patients often experience a great deal of difficulty in coming to terms with the new sensations and smells, the altered body image, bodily functions and body boundaries, and the long-term effects of having a stoma should never be under-estimated. As nurses are working with stoma patients' newly altered bodies, their approach, manner and the way in which they work with the body and the person, can considerably help patients in their processes of integrating the new experiences into their lives.

It is also important to learn personal strategies for dealing with embarrassment. Meerabeau (1999) concluded that nurses and doctors tend to use the same techniques for preventing embarrassment, such as 'matter of factness' and joking, but suggests that education programmes help practitioners and students to learn new and more supportive patterns of interaction.

Conclusion

Health workers, and particularly nurses, are potentially body workers *par excellence*. Body work can be challenging but by trying to understand the complexities and by working with patients through the transitions of their changing body and life experiences, nurses can develop strategies for effective body work. Working with patients and their bodies will present new challenges in the future. There are now more older people and the population is generally living longer, so issues of ageing and older age will require increasing attention. Disease patterns are changing in that there is now more chronic disease. In addition, technological and medical advances are increasingly preserving the lives of people severely injured, for example in road traffic accidents. We will need to understand the impact of chronic illness, severe traumatic injury and other disabilities on the human body but also of the embodied experience of those living with chronic illness or disability. The consumer culture in which we live will continue to bombard us with new messages and products to help us maintain healthy bodies. These new understandings may also need to be integrated into our knowledge and practice.

To conclude, Lawler (1991, p.227) suggests that

'nursing is in a unique if not ideal position from which to build a theory of the body, and from which to demonstrate the short-comings of positivist patterns of enquiry for such an enterprise . . .

nurses have a vast knowledge of the body . . . which is constructed in the context of a society in which people are taught to hide the body and some of its functions. While such a construction of the body continues, there will be social pressure to hide nursing and the work that nurses do, and by virtue of its privatised nature the body will also remain marginal in social science.'

References

Adams, T. & Keady, J. (2001) Why we need dementia care nursing. *Nursing Older People*, **13**, 2, 32–3.

Anderson, R. & Bury, M. (eds) (1988) *Living with Chronic Illness: the experience of patients and their families*. Unwin Hyman, London.

Bendelow, G.A. & Williams, S.J. (1998) Natural for women, abnormal for men: beliefs about pain and gender. In: S. Nettleton & J. Watson (eds) *The Body in Everyday Life*. Routledge, London.

Berger, P. & Luckman, T. (1967) *The Social Construction of Reality*. Penguin Books, Harmondsworth.

Blythway, B. & Johnson, J. (1998) The sight of age. In: S. Nettleton & J. Watson (eds) The *Body in Everyday Life*. Routledge, London.

Britton, C. (1998) 'Feeling let down': an exploration of an embodied sensation associated with breastfeeding. In: S. Nettleton (ed.) *The Body in Everyday Life*. Routledge, London.

Colton, H. (1983) *The Gift of Touch*. Sea View/Putnam, New York.

Descartes, R. (1986) *Discourse on Method and the Meditations* (trans. F.E. Sutcliffe). Penguin, Harmondsworth.

Dunnell, K. (1995) Are we healthier? *Population Trends*, **82**, 12–18.

Fairhurst, E. (1998) 'Growing old gracefully' as opposed to 'mutton dressed as lamb': the social construction of recognising older women. In: S. Nettleton & J. Watson (eds) *The Body in Everyday Life*. Routledge, London.

Featherstone, M. & Hepworth, M. (1991) The mask of ageing and the postmodern lifecourse. In: M. Featherstone, M. Hepworth & B.S. Turner (eds) *The Body: social processes and cultural theory*. Sage, London.

Fisher, L.M. & Joseph, D.H. (1989) A scale to measure attitudes about non-procedural touch. *Canadian Journal of Nursing Research*, **21**, 5–14.

Fraser, J. & Ross-Kerr, J. (1993) Psychophysiological effects of back massage on elderly institutionalised patients. *Journal of Advanced Nursing*, **18**, 238–45.

Giddens, A. (1991) *Modernity and Self-Identity: Self and society in the late modern age*. Polity Press, Cambridge.

Glaser, B.G. & Strauss, A.L. (1965) *Awareness of Dying*. Aldine Press, Chicago.

Goffman, E. (1969) *The Presentation of Self in Everyday Life*. Penguin, Harmondsworth.

Harre, R. (1986) Is the body a thing? *International Journal of Moral and Social Studies*, **1**, 3, 189–203.

Heath, H. (2002) *The outcomes of the work with Registered Nurses and Care Assistants with Older People in Nursing Homes*. Unpublished PhD Thesis, Brunel University.

Hepworth, M. & Featherstone, M. (1998) The male menopause: lay accounts and the cultural reconstruction of midlife. In: S. Nettleton & J. Watson (eds) *The Body in Everyday Life*. Routledge, London.

Kitwood, T. (1993a) Person and process in dementia. *International Journal of Geriatric Psychiatry*, **8**, 541–5.

Kitwood, T. (1993b) Discover the person – not the disease. *Journal of Dementia Care*, **1**, 1, 16–17.

Lawler, J. (1991) *Behind the Screens: Nursing, Somology and the Problem of the Body*. Churchill Livingstone, Melbourne.

Lawler, J. (1997) *The Body in Nursing*. Churchill Livingstone, Melbourne.

Leder, D. (1992) *The Body in Medical Thought and Practice*. Kluwer Academic, London.

le May, A. & Redfern, S. (1989) Touch and elderly people. In: J. Wilson Barnet & S. Robinson (eds) *Directions in Nursing Research*. Scutari, London.

Meerabeau, L. (1999) The management of embarassment and sexuality in health care. *Journal of Advanced Nursing*, **29**, 6, 1507–13.

Merleau-Ponty, M. (1962) *Phenomenology of Perception* (trans. C. Smith). Routledge & Kegan Paul, London.

Merleau-Ponty, M. (1964) The child's relations with others. In: J.M. Edie (ed.) *The Primary of Perception*, pp.96–155 (trans. W. Cobb). North Western University Press, Evanston.

Moore, J.R. & Gilbert, J.A. (1995) Elderly residents' perceptions of nurses' comforting touch. *Journal of Gerontological Nursing*, **21**, 6–13.

Nettleton, S. & Watson, J. (eds) (1998) *The Body in Everyday Life*. Routledge, London.

Price, B. (1990a) *Body Image, Nursing Concepts and Care*. Prentice-Hall, New York.

Price, B. (1990b) A model for body image care. *Journal of Advanced Nursing*, **15**, 585–93.

Sartre, J-P. (c. 1960) *Being and Nothingness*. Philosophical Library, New York.

Seymour, W. (1989) *Bodily Alterations: An introduction to a sociology of the body for health workers*. Allen and Unwin, Sydney.

Shilling, C. (1993) *The Body and Social Theory*. Sage, London.

Sontag, S. (1979) *Illness as Metaphor*. Vintage Books, New York.

Stutchfield, B. (2000) Stoma surgery in the older adult. *Elderly Care*, **11**, 10, 19–23.

Turner, B. (1984) *The Body in Society*. Basil Blackwell, Oxford.

Watson, J. (1998) Running around like a lunatic: Colin's body and the case of male embodiment. In: S. Nettleton & J. Watson (eds) *The Body in Everyday Life*. Routledge, London.

White, I. (1995) Controlling pain. In: H.B.M. Heath (ed.) *Foundations in Nursing Theory and Practice*. CV Mosby, London.

Williams, G. (1984) The genesis of chronic illness: narrative reconstructions. *Sociology of Health and Ilness*, **6**, 175–200.

Williams, S. (1996) The vicissitudes of embodiment across the chronic illness trajectory. *Body and Society*, **2**, 2, 23–47.

Williams, S. (1997) Modern medicine and the 'uncertain' body: from corporeality to hyperreality? *Social Science and Medicine*, **45**, 7, 1041–9.

Williams, B. & Barlow, J.H. (1998) Falling out of my shadow: lay perceptions of the body in the context of arthritis. In: S. Nettleton & J. Watson (eds) *The Body in Everyday Life*. Routledge, London.

Zola, I. (1973) Pathways to the doctor – from person to patient. *Social Science and Medicine*, Vol. 7. Pergamon Press, Oxford, pp.7–12.

Part 2
Sexuality Through the Lifespan

6. *Sexuality in Childhood and Adolescence*

Amanda Keighley

'Sexuality has always been a part of the human condition and people have always wished to understand it better.'

(Kirkendall, 1981, p.1)

Adults reflecting on how they developed their sexuality realise that different types of learning have taken place through experience and conditioning (Pates, 1992). There is the realisation that in expressing sexuality, we engage in the process of making and maintaining relationships. Sex not only refers to the physical act of intercourse or to feelings of sexual arousal, but can include reference to gender. In defining sexuality we must consider the physical, social, and cultural aspects of a person's life, all of which are interrelated (Woods, 1984). Sexuality involves the whole person and is a vital part of our being (Webb, 1985).

A chapter could be devoted to each of the aspects of sexuality. The intention here is to take a holistic approach to sexuality and the mind map (Buzan, 1995) in Fig. 1 represents a collection of thoughts around which to explore the theme of sexuality in the context of children and adolescents.

The importance of sexual health and its popularity as a topic for discussion in the media have not helped the development of concepts or definitions. Sexual health continues to mean different things to different people and this may indicate that an integrated approach to sexuality and sexual health could be the basis of a framework. This view is reinforced when a historical perspective is investigated (Allen, 1987).

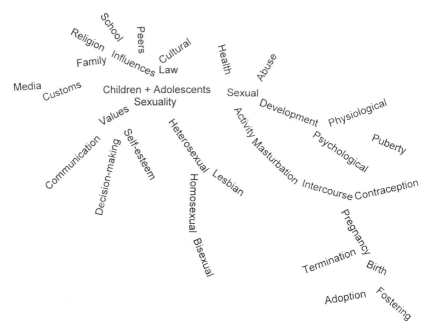

Fig. 6.1 Framework for sexuality.

Literature on children and adolescents

Sex education has been a part of the school curriculum since the 1930s. The original intention was to prevent illegitimacy (Barry, 1979). This changed over time with the 1960s and 1970s being primarily concerned with sex education and contraception. The 1980s saw the broadening of sex education into social education, relationships, values clarification and raising self-esteem (Reid, 1982). This was also reinforced by the World Health Organization which stated that the aim of sex education should be about 'understanding, mutual tenderness, delight and responsibility' (WHO, 1984).

The concept of having specific educational programmes to teach personal relationships and sexuality has been emphasised by developments and changes in legislation and policy in recent years. The Children Act 1989, *The Health of The Nation* (DoH, 1992) and *Sex Education in Schools* (DoH, 1994), each addressed the issue of sexuality for children and adolescents, fully or in part.

The Health of The Nation (DoH, 1992) made sexual health a priority and has resulted not only in other government initiatives (DoH, 1994), but also in voluntary organisations developing projects, such as the Family Planning Association's *Growing Up* series and the Brook Advisory Centre's Under 16s project (Brook Advisory Centre, 1993).

There seems to be little research that has looked in particular at adolescents in terms of their general health and illness (Bearinger & McAnarney, 1988). More recently the North American perspective has begun to alter with the introduction of specialist educational programmes looking at adolescent health. A similar picture is emerging in the United Kingdom, as adolescence becomes a focus in the work of general practitioners, psychiatrists, nurses, teachers and parents (Ferriman, 1995). A thread that runs through the literature is that of providing a seamless and community based service involving a multi-organisational approach in order to reach the maximum number of young people (Bearinger & Gephart, 1993; Brook Advisory Centre, 1993; Wong, 1995; Scott, 1995).

A deficit in the education and training of professionals is cited as the reason for the variability of service provision to meet the sexual health needs of children and adolescents. This is seen by some as an issue of role (Jackson, 1993a) and by others as a lack of knowledge and skills (Jackson, 1989; Jackson, 1991).

Studies in North America have evaluated sexual health programmes that have been undertaken in schools. The common objective of these studies has been the reduction of sexual risk-taking behaviour such as the frequency of intercourse, the non-use of contraception and the avoidance of sexually transmitted diseases (Kirby, 1992; Santelli & Beilenson, 1992; Kirby *et al.*, 1994).

Other studies have looked at related issues such as the relocation of the child or adolescent and its impact on their emotions and relationships (Puskar & Dvorsak, 1991), the needs of adolescent lesbians (Stine & Stevens-Simon, 1994) and the adolescent who is homeless and not attending school and the effect this has on their behaviour, including their sexual activity (Ragiel, 1994).

Studies looking at the sexual health of young people are also being undertaken in the United Kingdom (Jackson, 1993a; Jackson, 1993b; Bagnall, 1994; George, 1994; Gilbert, 1994; Shaw, 1995; Ellerby, 1997), spanning the health and education sectors. However, there are the questions of what is effective, how it is provided and by whom, together with the amount of service uptake need to be answered through larger studies, if an effective community service is to be provided to meet the sexual needs of children and adolescents.

The international literature reflects a wider picture of the issues surrounding the sexual health of children and adolescents. Studies have highlighted the general health needs including the sexuality of adolescents (Bearinger & Gephart, 1987; Baker *et al.*, 1994), the sexual education of children and adolescents (Van der Pligt & Richard, 1994), the evaluation of aspects of sexuality including sexual health programmes for children and adolescents (Bearinger, 1990; Males, 1993; Herold, 1994), the nature of sexual coercion as perceived by children and adolescents (Ogletree & Gast, 1993), the development of professional roles in meeting the sexual health needs of children and adolescents (Blum & Bearinger, 1990; Waterhouse & Metcalfe, 1991; Bearinger *et al.*, 1992; Ogletree & Gast, 1993; Iverson & Hays, 1994) and examples of good practice in meeting the sexual health needs of children and adolescents (Falsetti & Kovel, 1994; Lenderyou, 1996).

The literature would seem to indicate that we are becoming clearer about what it is we need to do as adults to enable children and adolescents to talk about feelings and relationships, but we are not consistent in our approach as either parents or professionals. Young people's 'chief sources of sex [sic] education are each other and the media' (Lenderyou, 1996, p.11).

Our behaviour and attitudes as adults towards sexuality ultimately have a consequence for children as they develop and

'seek to understand their sexual world, evidence of which is visibly present in their own bodies and in the members of their own family. Not only do they seek sexual knowledge but they strive to understand it, to make sense of it, and to do this they develop theories or hypotheses to explain what they observe.'
(Goldman & Goldman, 1982, p.6)

Beginning sexual development

When do children begin to develop their sexuality? Physiologically, a male baby will have erections within the first few days of being born and in a female baby there is vaginal lubrication within the first four to six hours following birth. Between the ages of two to six years Wolff (1973) describes the stage of '"primary identification" when children begin to compare themselves in size, age and sex with others, when they become aware of their own sexual identity and begin to model themselves on the parent of the same sex' (p.25). At this stage they also explore their own bodies, including their genitalia, and develop for the first time erotic feelings for the parent of the opposite sex, wishing for an exclusive relationship.

Masturbation is discouraged in many cultures, if not punished, from an early age. The disapproval from the parents forces the child to repress the natural beginnings of sexual activity, particularly when the child's behaviour is observed in a public place. For example, the three-year old boy who whilst out shopping with his mother, stands stroking his penis through his shorts. He is told to stop this behaviour. When he asks why, he is told that it is not nice to do that, to which he replies that it was.

According to Leung and Robson (1993), masturbation is considered to be normal behaviour, unless exhibited inappropriately or excessively, by children of all ages throughout the world. However, it continues to be denied by parents, who give the message that masturbation is dirty and abnormal. Unfortunately the result is that the child carries this view into adolescence and sometimes into adulthood. In extreme cases the effects of the parents' behaviour is generalised by their son or daughter, who then believes that any sexual behaviour including touching and kissing is highly damaging. It is little wonder that relationships, intimate or not, become dysfunctional and that confusion arises over information about safe sex. There have been mistaken diagnoses of epilepsy or abdominal pain in cases of masturbation in public. 'It is easy to understand the mistaken diagnosis when parents describe that their young child develops a glassy stare, becomes rigid or starts shaking as well as becoming pale and then drowsy' (Finkelstein *et al.*, 1996, p.324).

Masturbation is clearly more evident in boys as penile erections are easily recognised. The same is not the case with girls, who in order to achieve self-stimulation, engage in a variety of movements and body postures, which may well be misdiagnosed. The possible reason for this self-stimulatory behaviour has been cited as a reaction to family stresses such as divorce, death or parental absence. According to Finklestein *et al.* (1996), all the cases that reported episodes of masturbation stopped occurring in public over time. The only treatment had been the reassurance of the parents.

Children constantly ask questions, and it is important that these are answered honestly and realistically in order to stimulate further enquiry. However, this is less so when questions about sexuality arise, especially if this topic is mentioned in public, although at home the situation is more or less the same, with the replies being myth or just plain evasive. All of this contrives to foster a mystical cloud around the facts of life. The child perceives his or her questions to be subversive and acts to hide his or her behaviour. This is not an example of maladaptive behaviour on the part of the child. Rather 'sexual curiosity … finds expression in general curiosity about the world. The sexual drive is transformed into an urge to learn' (Wolff, 1973, p.42).

Sexual development may also be dysfunctional. From birth there are a number of physical manifestations that will impact on the development of the individual with one of the following conditions.

- An abnormality in the sex chromosomes can result in a profound effect not only on the sexual characteristics but in the physical health and psychological development of the individual. In males, an extra sex chromosome will result in Klinefelter's syndrome. Men with this condition do not develop secondary sex characteristics. They have poorly developed muscle, enlarged breasts and are infertile because of an inability to produce sperm. They also tend to have mild learning disability.
- Women who have only one, instead of two, sex chromosomes are diagnosed with Turner syndrome. The development of the external genitalia is normal, but the ovaries do not develop or function normally and they are therefore infertile. Women with this condition are not obviously distinguishable from the rest of the female population, except that they tend to be shorter in stature and may also have a mild learning disability.
- Hormonal errors can also occur during pregnancy, resulting in hermaphroditism. The individual is born with both testicular and ovarian tissue. They may have one gonad of each gender (one testicle and one ovary) or a combination of both types of tissue. True hermaphroditism is rare. It is pseudohermaphroditism that is the more common condition. Here the individual has either testes or ovaries, which match their chromosomal gender. The hormonal error affects the external genitalia and sometimes the internal reproductive organs. Either they are ambiguous or may resemble those of the opposite gender.

These conditions question the notion of gender identity and how it is established, with most of the research being undertaken by examining the experiences of pseudohermaphrodites. The results of the studies highlight the complexity of the interface between biological and psychological factors, with researchers emphasising one or other of the factors, thereby continuing the nature–nurture debate (Nevid *et al.*, 1995).

Cultural influences

It is also suggested (Goldman & Goldman, 1982) that in western cultures, girls are encouraged by their mothers to be less assertive and aggressive than their brothers. It would seem that the stereotyping of the genders continues to exist in a covert way. Goldman and Goldman (1982) continue the premise 'that culture strongly influences sexual behaviour' (p.8), and that differing cultures may follow different 'strategies in sexual thinking and achieve varying levels of knowledge and insight about sex at differing ages' (Goldman & Goldman, 1982, p.8).

Child rearing practices, however similar or dissimilar, provide both a positive and negative cognitive framework within which a child has to function. Religion and sexual morality are often viewed by religious groups as being closely linked if not actually congruent. Programmes in religious education frequently emphasise the one as a basis for the other. However there is very little literature on the relationship between religious and sexual thinking. What is acknowledged is the theoretical relationships between religion, morality and sexuality (Fraser, 1972).

Cultural differences are also significant. For example, adolescents from Asian or Arab cultures are now the third or fourth generation of families who have settled in the UK. They find themselves experiencing the interface between their own culture and that of the country in which they are living. This can create conflicts including how sexual development takes place, e.g. the parents' right to withdraw their child from sex education in school. The adolescent then finds another way to access that information, probably through their peer group. Getting to know members of the opposite sex can take place through meeting in public places, such as shops. This demonstrates how adolescents from different cultures find ways of accessing information and of behaving that are not viewed as being in direct conflict with their own culture.

At the time of writing, Fraser's (1972) observation that sexuality in children remains relatively unresearched still holds true. Childhood innocence continues to be equated with sexual innocence and there is a reluctance to identify sexuality as part of a child's development before the onset of puberty. This is reinforced by the work of Freud, specifically his theory of latency, which Fraser (1972) views as adding to the concept of child sexuality not being explored, except in the area of child abuse. This would seem to indicate that the insight into only part of the picture of children and sexuality is an extremely negative one.

Sexual exploitation

Sexual abuse damages children both physically and psychologically, as a child is not ready for a sexual relationship. The con-

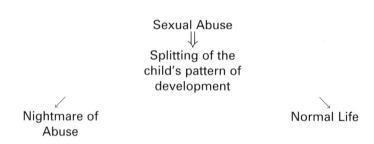

Figure 6.2 Splitting the child's normal development.

sequence for the child is the splitting of their normal development (see Fig. 2).

The nightmare of sexual abuse is filed away in the mind of the child. If the child is unable to tell of the abuse, then there is a possibility that later on in life a trigger, for example a sexual relationship with a boy- or a girlfriend, will release feelings of devastation. These feelings may well be overwhelming together with being at some level out of touch with reality.

Sexual abuse has been specifically defined as 'the exploitation of a child for sexual gratification' (Winkley, 1996, p.209). Sexual contact can take varying forms, from inappropriate fondling to full intercourse. It is important that as professionals we do not collude in incidents of child sexual abuse in a bid to avoid facing the emotional impact on those concerned and ourselves.

Child sexual abuse has the greatest impact of any type of abuse and affects the child's normal development. The consequence for sexually abused children is the increased risk of developing mental health problems in adulthood (Mullen, 1990). There is a need to take seriously the accounts of children who complain of sexual abuse. They rarely lie, with about 98% of children telling the truth (Jones & McQuiston, 1989). What also needs to be recognised is that delay in acknowledging and acting on children's accounts is a major feature in child sex abuse. This heightens the impact of the feelings of shame and guilt that are involved, where the child feels that the abuse was their fault, although this is not the case. The child will rarely directly tell others, having been bribed or threatened to remain quiet. In some cases the child will confide in a friend who may then seek out an adult for help.

The sexually abused child develops the ability to adapt to the situation in which they are being abused, but at great cost to themselves. Their loss of self-esteem and the feeling of being a victim can become established. The child continues to have to face a situation from which there is no escape. All this produces high stress levels resulting in learned helplessness (Peterson & Seligman, 1983).

Types of sexual abuse

Anal abuse is common in younger girls and boys, with a third of all sexually abused children under five years of age, while in girls aged between six and ten years, vaginal abuse is increasingly more common. More than half of the children who are abused have no physical signs on examination, as they have been subjected to masturbation, oral sex, fondling or pornography.

The perpetrator is usually someone who the child knows and who has actively 'targeted and groomed this child for abuse' (Winkley, 1996, p.211). The majority of perpetrators of sexual abuse are male adults, but boys of between six to seven years are increasingly guilty of abusing another child. There is also a significant minority of female abusers, often the mother.

Recognising child sex abuse, assessing and linking the information together to make a 'reliable diagnosis requires an experienced professional team approach' (Winkley, 1996, p.221). Many professionals who come into contact with children, such as nurses, teachers, health visitors and doctors may be alerted to the signs of child sex abuse; for example, younger children who suddenly behave in a sexually inappropriate manner by constantly masturbating, or by hinting about abuse. Older children may abuse themselves using drugs or alcohol, or run away to escape the abusive environment.

The symptoms that a sexually abused child may present with are localised injury or infection around the area of abuse, inappropriate sexual knowledge or a change in behaviour. A change in the behaviour of a child is sometimes ignored as it is perceived as 'acting out' or 'attention seeking'. The psychological effects of abuse may be the clue to what the child is experiencing and may manifest themselves as anxiety, eating or sleeping disorders, withdrawal, depression, aggression, temper tantrums, drug and alcohol misuse, prostitution and suicide. 'There is a recognised association between sexual abuse as a child and outcomes such as pregnancy in adolescence, prostitution and anorexia' (Winkley, 1996, p.214).

Role of the professional

Once signs of child sex abuse are suspected it is important that the warning signs, dates, times and what the child says and does are clearly documented. In gaining clarification, do not put words into the child's mouth. Allow the child time to express both what has happened and how they feel about the situation. This can be done verbally and/or through the use of drawing as a vehicle for the child telling their story. Symbolism is a valuable resource to use with children, enabling them to be clear about what it is that they wish to convey as they explain their pictures (Woolfson, 1982; Lewis & Greene, 1983; Yates *et al.*, 1985; Martin, 1994). During these sessions it is important to elicit from the child the whereabouts of any hurt or pain.

Collecting evidence of this nature when the child is ready is vitally important, because as a result of this action the child may subsequently be threatened and therefore say nothing at a later date. Another consideration is that the abusing relationship may exist between more than two parties and that the family is sexually abusive.

It would be easy to assume that only those professionals who work directly with children need to be aware of the child protection guidelines and procedures. This is not the case. Working with one or more members of a family may bring to light issues of child abuse in a number of contexts as 'child maltreatment is determined by forces at work in the individual, the family and in the community and culture in which the individual and family are embedded' (Vinson *et al.*, 1996, p.523). It is imperative to remember that the protection of the child always comes first.

Development of sexual knowledge

The development of sex education for children and adolescents is a worldwide phenomenon, with agreement that they need to be informed about sexual matters. The controversy emerges over the following questions (Fraser, 1972): whose responsibility is it, school or home; at what age should the teaching begin; and what is suitable for inclusion in the content?

It would seem that if, like Goldman and Goldman (1982), we view the whole picture then Fraser's comment can be seen in context. The slow development of sex determination seems to be influenced by several factors. These are first, the process of explanations, which is difficult as it requires the child to function at a high level of operational thinking and thereby be able to hypothesise. Second, the child needs to develop 'scientific realism' which can be provided through, 'sequential lessons in human biology. All of this is rarely experienced before the age of fifteen years' (Goldman & Goldman, 1982, p.8).

Education about sexuality requires young people to develop self-esteem, as this leads them to 'feel positive about themselves, they are more likely to develop non exploitive, caring relationships, and are themselves less likely to be exploited by others' (The Clarity Collective, 1989, p.1). Learning is an exploration, where knowledge is acquired and contextualised. Children under the age of eight relate most of what they learn to themselves and their individual experience (Tonks, 1996). Sexual information must then be age-appropriate and not be seen as preparing children for every possible sexual encounter. Throughout the first 12 years of their lives children will learn formally and informally about a range of topics that are all linked to sexuality and relationships. The identification of these links may not be made, as was borne out by the research where 'We were aware that a straightforward question about sex education in primary schools might not give a very full response ... partly because teenagers – and their parents – might not have interpreted what they were being taught as "sex education"' (Allen, 1987, p.7). The topics that were covered in primary school were:

- talking or going with strangers
- changes in boys'/girls' bodies
- animal reproduction
- human reproduction
- family/parenthood.

The person who delivers the information and the context in which they do so stays with the child; for example, talking to or going with strangers is an issue of safety and may well be talked through by a member of the local police. Animal and human reproduction will have been covered during the science part of the curriculum and therefore be seen by the children as a process that happens, but is difficult for them to relate to their own experience, unless they are part of an animal farming community. 'It was very striking how little parents appeared to know about the education given in primary schools about changes in boys' and girls' bodies' (Allen, 1987, p.10).

It would seem that the points to remember as professionals when involved with children are that:

- information should be age-appropriate
- a lack of response may be due to the fact that what is being taught is beyond the child's ability

- there is a correlation between a child having a low level of anxiety and being most at risk
- clear and accurate communication is paramount between the parties involved including the child.

Adolescent sexuality

Adolescence spans the age range from twelve to twenty. During this period sexuality is a major development that is marked by the physical, psychological and social changes of adolescence (Wong, 1995). Puberty is the most obvious part of this development, with changes occurring over a time span of four to five years. These include the growth spurt, 'feeling all arms and legs', alterations in body shape such as the development of genitalia and breasts, menstruation or ejaculation, spots, and voice breaking in boys. All of these changes have a marked impact on the way in which adolescents perceive their bodies. The parallel development of sexual feelings and cognitive skills may result in dissonance – am I normal feeling this way? – do I look okay? Self-esteem can seem to falter. The development of formal operational thinking and the increased ability to make decisions enable the adolescent to cope with issues of sexuality. Giving adolescents new information about sexual matters is a matter of straightforward understanding of their needs. The challenge is how far are we able to influence them in relation to their levels of risk taking and subsequent behaviour.

In general adolescents agree that learning about sexual development is required, but feel that it is often too little too late and biased towards a biological input (Prendergast, 1993; Lenderyou, 1996). Feeling isolated and unable to talk to anyone, including their parents, about personal issues, the experience can be worse for boys (Lenderyou, 1996) and worse still for homosexual and bisexual adolescents (Epstein, 1994).

Adolescents' development of a sexual identity is marked by the separation of their own emotional and social identities from those of their families. The formation of close relationships with same-sex peers is a feature the social life of young adolescents, who may experiment sexually with these peers in order to satisfy their curiosity. At this stage relationships with the opposite sex are maintained at a distance, with about one third of males and one quarter of females having experienced sexual intercourse by the age of 15 (Wong, 1995). It is this proportion of adolescents who are at high risk in terms of behaviour problems and sexually transmitted diseases (Seidman & Rieder, 1994) (see Chapter 12).

The middle and late years of adolescence see couples pairing off and intimate relationships developing, although the degree of intimacy varies. According to Wong (1995, p.837), 'adolescents find it hard to believe that sex can exist without love'. Relationships during adolescence have a strong emotional attachment and are also a time when adolescents question their sexual orientation (which sex a person is attracted to) through uncertainty. There will be those who have identified themselves as homosexual, lesbian or bisexual. Development for these groups occurs over a long period and has been described as an unsure backwards and forwards movement, rather than a steady progression (Coleman & Remafedi, 1989).

The pivot of adolescence is puberty, but this is more than a series of physical manifestations. Adolescence is a period of development that takes time and requires support by parent figures. The lack of this means that 'the adolescents must make a jump to a false maturity and lose their greatest asset: freedom to have ideas and to act on impulse' (Winnicott, 1971, pp.149–50).

Adults, whether parents or professionals, tend to be uncomfortable talking with adolescents about sexuality and personal relationships, believing that young people will find out for themselves. This misguided notion results in adolescents relying on their peers and the media. The latter source is now far more acceptable. Health education experts view teenage magazines as having a vital role in providing accurate information and advice that is presented in a format acceptable to adolescents (Fisher, 1997). However, the vast majority of this material is aimed at girls and is not interactive, therefore any questions that the adolescent might have go unanswered.

Sexual activity is more than a series of mechanical processes beginning with intercourse and ending in pregnancy and or disease. Adolescents want to know how to practise safe sex through being assertive and saying no, through to what forms of contraception are available. They also need to know the facts about sexually transmitted diseases (STDs), as 'nearly all STDs are contracted through behaviours that can be avoided or modified' (Hale & Trumbetta, 1996, p.109).

Role of the professionals

As professionals we may not be involved on a regular basis in advising on sexual health and sex education to children and adolescents. What we may be engaged in are sporadic interventions involving children and adolescents, which require us to offer support, advice, information and education. Whatever the level of contact we must ensure that we are effective. The following four points have been highlighted when evaluating the effectiveness of sexual health and sex education programmes (Few *et al.*, 1996, p.3). Such programmes should

- promote the active involvement of children in learning
- be appropriate to the age of the child
- increase self-esteem
- promote the development of skills and positive attitudes to sexual health.

It must be remembered that sexuality is one part of children's and adolescents' maturity and cannot be separated from other cognitive and social development. This is particularly important for boys (Davidson, 1990) as there is an increased awareness of their needs in the broader context of education, including sexual and mental health.

As professionals we need to be comfortable with our own sexuality. We too need to explore our attitudes towards sexuality and thereby gain confidence when talking to others, including children and adolescents. For example, what do we think about sexual preferences different to our own? Are we aware of when the process of sexuality increases and decreases throughout the life cycle? Once we have gained insight into ourselves, then we are more able to discuss sexuality with other people, e.g. a partner, friends or colleagues.

Communicating effectively is important as often children and adolescents do not make clear what it is they wish to discuss. Active listening is the first step; do not feel the need to question at this stage, otherwise the child or adolescent may feel intimidated and stop talking. You may also feel uncomfortable with what has been said and find yourself questioning aspects of your own sexuality. It is difficult not to allow your own values to influence your reactions, especially when faced with what you may consider to be inappropriate behaviour, such as sexual promiscuity which may challenge your traditional views, or having your liberal views challenged by very traditional views on sexuality.

A child or adolescent may decide that you are the person with whom they wish to share their feelings about their sexuality. Their expectation will very likely be veiled in fear – fear of the unknown. Underneath this will be the hope of being listened to and not judged, being able to seek advice and enabled to make their own decisions and treated with respect. Do not promise a child or an adolescent absolute confidentiality and never break that restricted confidentiality without first informing them. We must also recognise our own limitations and know when and to whom to refer.

How we as practitioners work with children and adolescents around issues of sexual health may make us reflect on the need to update our own knowledge and skills. Sexuality, like communication, is an aspect of our lives that we can all demonstrate. The degree to which we are skilled and effective not only depends on our knowledge and skills but also our self-awareness about our own sexuality. Contact with children and adolescents does not necessarily make any of us competent to talk through issues of sexual health or sex education. What it does offer is the opportunity to explore this part of human development for ourselves in a sensitive and supported way, which in turn we may be able to share with the children and adolescents with whom we work.

References

Allen, I. (1987) *Education in Sex and Personal Relationships*. Policy Studies Institute, London.

Bagnall, P. (1994) Investing in school-age children's health. *Nursing Times*, **90**, 31, 27–9.

Baker, J., Hutchinson, G., Miles, B., Ower, H. & Tonkin, K. (1994) Sexuality in adolescents. *Journal of Australian Paediatric Nursing*, **5**, 1, 23–6.

Barry, S.M.K. (1979) Sex education in its curricular context: the evaluation of a sex education programme in Borehamwood schools with a view to assessing its contribution to the development of 'social maturity'. PhD thesis, Brunel University. In: I. Allen (ed.), *Education in Sex and Personal Relationships*. Policy Studies Institute, London.

Bearinger, L.H. (1990) Study group report on the impact of television on adolescent views of sexuality. *Journal of Adolescent Health Care*, **11**, 71–5.

Bearinger, L.H. & Gephart, J. (1987) Priorities for adolescent health: recommendations of a national conference. *The American Journal of Maternal/Child Nursing*, **12**, May/June, 161–4.

Bearinger, L.H. & McAnarney, E.R. (1988) Integrated community health delivery programs for youth. *Journal of Adolescent Health Care*, **9**, 36S–40S.

Bearinger, L.H., Gephart, J. & Blum, R.W. (1992) Nursing competence in adolescent health: anticipating the future needs of youth. *Journal of Professional Nursing*, **8**, 2, 80–86.

Bearinger, L.H. & Gephart, J. (1993) Interdisciplinary education in adolescent health. *Journal of Paediatric Health*, **29**[suppl.] 1, S10–S15.

Blum, R.W. & Bearinger, L.H. (1990) Knowledge and attitudes of health professionals towards adolescent health care. *Journal of Adolescent Health Care*, **11**, 289–94.

Brook Advisory Centre (1993) *Under 16s Project*. Department of Health, London.

Brown, L. (ed.) (1981) *Sex Education in the Eighties*. Plenum Press, New York.

Buzan, T. (1995) *Use Your Head*. BBC Books, London.

Coleman & Remafedi (1989) In: D. Epstein (1994) *Challenging Lesbian and Gay Inequalities in Education*. Open University Press, Buckingham.

Davidson, N. (1990) *Boys Will Be ... Sex Education and Young Men*. Bedford Square Press, London.

Department of Health (1992) *The Health of The Nation*. DoH, London.

Department of Health (1994) *Sex Education in Schools*. DoH, London.

Ellerby, K. (1997) Contraception and safer sex. *Practice Nursing*, **8**, 8, 16–19.

Epstein, D. (1994) *Challenging Lesbian and Gay Inequalities in Education*. Open University Press, Buckingham.

Falsetti, D. & Kovel, A. (1994) How one school based clinic is meeting the challenge of adolescent health care. *Journal of the American Academy of Nurse Practitioners*, **6**, 8, 363–8.

Family Planning Association (1993) *Growing Up Series*. Department of Health, London.

Ferriman, A. (1995) Healthfront. Teenage problems. *Daily Telegraph Magazine*, 7 Oct., 59.

Few, C., Hicken, I. & Butterworth, T. (1996) *Principles and Practices of Sexual Health and Sex Education in Schools*. University of Manchester Press, Manchester.

Finkelstein, E., Amichai, B., Jaworowski, S. & Mukamel, M. (1996) Masturbation in prepubescent children: a case report and review of the literature. *Child: Care, Health and Development*, **22**, 5, 323–6.

Fisher, F. (1997) Teenage hotline. *Nursing*, **11**, 41, 19.

Fraser, S.E (ed.) (1972) *Sex, Schools and Society*. Anrora, New York.

George, M. (1994) Healthy sexuality. *Nursing Standard*, **8**, 50, 21–22.

Gilbert, S. (1994) Is the message getting across? *Professional Nurse*, Aug., 765–9.

Goldman, R. & Goldman, J. (1982) *Children's Sexual Thinking*. Routledge & Kegan Paul, London.

Hale, P.J. & Trumbetta, S.L. (1996) Women's self-efficacy and sexually transmitted disease preventative behaviours. *Research in Nursing and Health*, **19**, 101–10.

Herold, E.S. (1994) Teenage sexuality and sexual health. *Canadian Journal of Public Health*, **8**, 4, 223–4.

Hobbs, T. (1992) *Experiential Training*. Routledge, London.

Iverson, C.J. & Hays, B.J. (1994) School nursing in the 21st century: prediction and readiness. *Journal of School Nursing*, **10**, 4, 19–24.

Jackson, D. (1989) Sex education in Halton secondary schools. *School Nurse*, **62**, 7, 219–21.

Jackson, D. (1991) HIV/AIDS: getting the message across. *Health Visitor*, **64**, 7, 212.

Jackson, D. (1993a) Fighting for the future. *Health Visitor*, **66**, 5, 159–60.

Jackson, D. (1993b) Fax of life. *Health Visitor*, **66**, 8, 293–4.

Jones, D. & McQuiston, M. (1989) *Interviewing the Sexually Abused Child*. Gaskell, London.

Kirby, D. (1992) School based programs to reduce sexual risk-taking behaviors. *Journal of School Health*, **62**, 7, 280–87.

Kirby, D., Short, L., Collins, J., *et al.* (1994) School-based programs to reduce sexual risk behaviors: a review of effectiveness. *Public Health Reports*, **109**, 3, 339–60.

Kirkendall, L.A. (1981) Sex education in the United States. In: L. Brown (ed.) (1981) *Sex Education in the Eighties*. Plenum Press, New York.

Lenderyou, G. (1996) What's the big secret? *Children UK*, Winter, 11.

Leung, A.K.C. & Robson, W.L. (1993) Childhood masturbation. *Clinical Paediatrics*, **32**, 238–41.

Lewis, D. & Greene, J. (1983) *Your Child's Drawings . . . Their Hidden Meaning*. Hutchinson, London.

Males, M. (1993) School-age pregnancy: why hasn't prevention worked? *Journal of School Health*, **63**, 10, 429–32.

Martin, J. (1994) A channel from the subconscious. *Professional Nurse*, October, 14–19.

Mullen, P.E. (1990) The long term effects of child sexual assault on the mental health of victims. *Journal of Forensic Psychiatry*, **1**, 13–34.

Nevid, J.S., Fichner-Rathus, L. & Rathus, S.A. (1995) *Human Sexuality in a World of Diversity* (second edition). Allyn & Bacon, Boston.

Ogletree, R.J. & Gast, J. (1993) Female adolescent sexual coercion: implications for health educators. *Journal of Health Education*, **24**, 4, 203–208.

Pates, R. (1992) An Introduction to working with sexuality. In: T. Hobbs (ed.) *Experiental Training*. Routledge, London.

Peterson, C. & Seligman, M. (1983) Learned helplessness and victimisation. *Journal of Social Issues*, **39**, 103–16.

Prendergast, S. (1993) *This is the Time to Grow Up: Girls' experience of menstruation in school*. Health Promotion Research Trust, Cambridge.

Puskar, K.R. & Dvorsak, K.G. (1991) Relocation stress in adolescents: helping teenagers cope with a moving dilemma. *Paediatric Nursing*, **17**, 3, 295–8.

Ragiel, C. (1994) Critique of lifestyles, adaptive strategies and sexual behaviors of homeless adolescents. *Nursing Scan in Research*, **7**, 2, 14.

Reid, D. (1982) School sex education and the causes of unintended teenage pregnancies: a review. *Health Education Journal*, **41**, 1, 4–10.

Santelli, J.S. & Beilenson, P. (1992) Risk factors for adolescent sexual behavior, fertility and sexually transmitted diseases. *Journal of School Health*, **62**, 7, 271–9.

Scott, J. (1995) School's out . . . for family planning. *Nursing Standard*, **9**, 45, 20–21.

Seidman, S. & Rieder, R. (1994) A review of sexual behaviour in the United States. *American Journal of Psychiatry*, **151**, 3, 330–41.

Shaw, S. (1995) Teen health on record. *Primary Health Care*, **5**, 8, 31–3.

Stine, K. & Stevens-Simon, C. (1994) Lesbians also need attention as adolescents. *Nurse Practitioner: American Journal of Primary Health Care*, **19**, 5, 21.

The Children Act (1989). HMSO, London.

The Clarity Collective (1989) *Taught not Caught: Strategies for Sex Education* (second edition). LDA, Cambridgeshire.

Tonks, D. (1996) *Teaching Aids*. Routledge, London.

Van der Pligt, J. & Richard, R. (1994) Changing adolescents' sexual behaviour: perceived risk, self-efficacy and anticipated regret. *Journal of Patient Education and Counselling*, **23**, 3, 187–96.

Vinson, T. (1996) Neighbourhoods, networks and child abuse. *British Journal of Social Work*, **26**, 4, 523.

Waterhouse, J. & Metcalfe, M. (1991) Attitudes towards nurses discussing sexual concerns with patients. *Journal of Advanced Nursing*, **16**, 1048–54.

Webb, C. (1985) *Sexuality, Nursing and Health*. John Wiley, New York.

Whaley, L.L. & Wong, D.L. (1995) *Nursing Care of Infants and Children* (fifth edition). C V Mosby, St Louis.

WHO Regional Office for Europe (1984) *Family planning and sex education of young people*. World Health Organization, Geneva.

Winkley, L. (1996) *Emotional Problems in Children and Young People*. Cassell, London.

Winnicott, D.W. (1971) *Playing and Reality*. Tavistock/Routledge, London.

Wolff, S. (1973) *Children Under Stress*. Pelican, London.

Wong, D.L. (1995) Health promotion of the adolescent and family. In: L.L. Whaley & D.L. Wong (eds). *Nursing Care of Infants and Children* (fifth edition). C V Mosby, St Louis.

Woods, N.F. (1984) *Human Sexuality in Health and Illness*. C V Mosby, St Louis.

Woolfson, R. (1982) Interpretation of drawings. *Times Educational Supplement*, 19 November.

Yates, A., Beutler, L.E. & Crago, M. (1985) Drawings by child victims of incest. *Child Abuse and Neglect*, **9**, 183–9.

106

7. Sexuality and People with a Learning Disability

Amanda Keighley

Making and maintaining relationships is a complex activity. It affects us all as the media constantly bombards us, telling us how to handle our relationships. This, together with personal experience and formal education, enables us to come to terms with our own sexuality: 'None of us makes our life alone' (O'Brien, 1987, p.175).

To develop our life experiences we rely on both formal and informal learning. Both these strands must be identified, take place, be assimilated within a structure and delivered through a system or framework. The formal approach is usually met via school and other avenues of education, such as part-time college courses. The informal approach takes place within the family and peer group settings. The framework for the latter can be loose or seemingly non-existent, making it difficult to meet the needs of those individuals who have a learning disability. People with a learning disability (PWLD) are vulnerable, particularly when they have to deal with the major challenges of making and maintaining relationships at all levels, including those that are of an intimate and/or sexual nature.

Before exploring the potentially tricky path of helping people with a learning disability to make and maintain relationships, it would seem prudent to look at a historical overview. Society's attitudes to people with a learning disability have dictated and continue to dictate how this group will be viewed by society, including their expression of their sexuality.

Historical overview

The history surrounding people with a learning disability tends either to be concerned with legal and institutional landmarks or to

107

deal with scientific discoveries and educational reforms. There is little social history to refer to: individuals with a learning disability tend to be hidden away even in historical accounts.

Prior to the late eighteenth century, discussions relating to idiocy, – as learning disability was then known – are fragmentary. Those that remain show a preoccupation with human status and their origins. The views of Paracelsus in the sixteenth century that idiots do not suffer from worldly corruption to the extent of the rest of society, being perpetual children and a natural element of a society which accepted them, were still one viewpoint. The other recurrent theme in the Christian world at this time was based on the perspective of St Augustine of Hippo, who viewed the existence of people with a learning disability as a consequence of the evils of mankind. The notion that people with a learning disability were subhuman and without a soul pervaded up until the end of the nineteenth century.

In unique contrast to the subhuman theory, descriptions given by outside observers upon cretins in the Swiss Alps are positive, if somewhat romantic. (Cretinism is the result of low levels or the absence of the hormone thyroxin in the developing child.) Due to the mineral content in the drinking water in certain parts of the Alps, cretinism was common. These individuals were regarded by the Swiss valley inhabitants as ' "heavenly beings"; incapable of sin; and a blessing to their families' (Coxe, 1779). It is not known why this group of people was viewed so positively. What does become apparent is the need to understand clearly the social basis of attitudes. This is vital to any overall comprehension of 'idiocy'.

The organic cause of idiocy was not really looked at until the twentieth century, when social categories of 'defectives' were devised. The discovery that mental deficiency was related to genetic defects was also a twentieth century phenomenon. The understanding of this new science was limited, as mental defectives were still viewed as representing the evils of society, which they had inherited from their parents. Tredgold (1908) emphasised this point on heredity stating that 90% of all mental defectives were the result of defects inherent in germinal plasm.

The Victorians, who believed that such people were uncivilised and particularly prone to sin, now promoted the image of mental defectives as animals. Having once been an animal to be pitied, the mental defective now became a danger, a degenerate of the human race. It was the idiots who were alcoholics, thieves, the result of poverty and illegitimacy. This indiscriminate linking of mental defectives with social problems became commonplace. For example, a pressure group was formed in 1896 called the National Association for the Care and the Control of the Feeble Minded. It called for the lifetime segregation of defectives, with particular emphasis on the prevention of sexuality and reproduction. This view was upheld by the middle classes in the face of the working classes' fertility, and was reinforced further by the scaremongering about a 'brain drain' in Britain by the Eugenics Society. Their belief fostered the 'anxieties that if their [PWLD] sexuality were not suppressed the handicapped would prolifically reproduce or engage in uncontrollable bursts of sexual violence' (Elwood, 1981, p.169).

Myths

Historically, people with a learning disability have often been ignored. If it is recognised, their sexuality tends to be surrounded by myth, although Koegel and Whittemore (1983) take the view that many of these have now disappeared. The assumption of sexual aggression in men with a learning disability who display behaviour such as urinating in public or walking around with their flies undone is fallacious, as these are not acts of sexual perversion, but arise from ignorance and a lack of social skills (Elwood, 1981). Another myth has been that masturbation will cause physical damage – 'you'll go blind ... it'll make you deaf'.

Myths even surround the educational component of sexuality. These include the withholding of information about sexuality as a deterrent from sexual activity, and the belief that sex education will entice people with a learning disability to engage in sexual activity. Neither is accurate. Those educating this particular group about issues of sexuality need to consider the level at which the material is being presented, and should not take a retrospective approach in which the material is tackled only when the person concerned has had the experience. For example, if the topic of menstruation is addressed once a young woman has begun to menstruate such an approach may result in emotional distress for the individual.

Values

'The process by which we discern what is good or humanising is underpinned by our moral values. In the context of sexuality there will be sexual–moral values, which serve as points of reference in evaluation, decision making or action.'

(Morris, 1994, p.xix)

Moral growth is reinforced through the interplay of accepting and challenging in an environment that is willing to be non-judgmental and accept a person's values and way of being. The statement from the United Nations (1971) that people with a learning disability have the same rights further supports this. In defining sexual health the World Health Organization is clear as to the boundaries, both individually and as part of a culture:

> 'A capacity to enjoy and control sexual and reproductive behaviour in accordance with a social and personal ethic. Freedom from fear, shame, guilt, false belief and other psychological factors inhibiting sexual response and impairing sexual relationships and freedom from organic disorders, diseases and deficiencies that interfere with sexual and reproductive functions.'
>
> (WHO, 1986)

The virtuous tone of these pronouncements does not, however, necessarily mean that they are having the desired effect. Only low numbers of women with learning disability are taking up the breast and cervical screening services (Pearson *et al.*, 1998; Robinson, 1998; Taylor *et al.*, 1998). And the wider picture shows that not everyone accepts the United Nation's Declaration of Rights for People with a Learning Disability (Carr, 1995).

Vulnerability

Lack of knowledge about their personal rights leaves people with a learning disability vulnerable to sexual abuse. They are also vulnerable to the message that they must always conform to the wishes of others, which leads them to follow and obey, unable to say no in situations where there is a risk of illegal activity and exploitation. Sobsey (1994, p.94) highlights an 'emerging body of research linking disability with sexual abuse and assault...' which '...leaves little doubt that the problem is a severe one'. He goes on to comment that 'little information is available to clarify the nature of the link between disability and sexual victimisation'. Sobsey (1994) argues that the link between a person's disability and dependence with an increased risk of abuse has little by way of research to support such a view. The research that has been undertaken (Belsky, 1980; Garbarino & Stocking, 1980) suggests that society's response to disability may be more important than the disability itself in increasing

110

vulnerability and may imply that intervention must be aimed primarily at systems rather than individuals.

Often the relationship between a carer and someone with a learning disability can become one of power and control for the carer. While this may seem a more obvious consequence within a residential or day service, it can also feature within a family setting. There is also a greater risk that men will commit sexual offences against women (Turk & Brown, 1993) and that women 'are more likely to put themselves at risk by difficult or overt sexual behaviour' (Brown & Barrett, 1994, p.57). This reflects the relative power of both men and women with learning disabilities, and highlights the vulnerability of women and men who are subject to sexual abuse, particularly when the learning disability is of a profound level. It is recognised that people with a profound learning disability do have sexual needs and drives, but the nature of the behaviour may be self-harming, such as rubbing the genitalia against a hard surface. Their behaviour may also leave them open to being preyed upon by others and being unable to defend themselves (Reid, 1995).

Clarifying sexual motivation

There are over 800 cases of abuse reported each year in England and Wales involving people with a learning disability, with specific figures of over 40% being committed by people with a learning disability (Gaze, 1992). It could be construed, albeit inaccurately, from this information that people with a learning disability are more likely to commit such offences than the rest of the population. However, as Fenwick (1994) argues, rather than just focusing on the numbers of people with a learning disability who are abused or who have perpetrated abuse, attention should be re-focused on whether the behaviours that are exhibited are sexually motivated. Services are likely to construe behaviours as sexual on a rather haphazard basis, just as they compound the problem by labelling behaviours 'difficult' more or less randomly (Brown & Barrett, 1994).

Whether a behaviour is sexually motivated needs to be clarified. The work of Brown and Barrett (1994) offers a number of approaches:

- the ABC (antecedent, behaviour, and consequence) chart
- counselling and psychotherapy
- O'Brien's Five Accomplishments (presence, choice, competence, respect and participation).

The common thread in any approach is the need for a systematic method, which can begin to develop a holistic picture of behaviour that is either sexually motivated or is a result of other trauma or experiences.

The ABC chart

The ABC represents three components which offer a framework in which behaviours are viewed in the context of what has taken place immediately before, the behaviour itself and what has taken place immediately after the behaviour has been observed.

A: What is happening immediately before the behaviour. Are there signs that the person is sexually aroused?
B: The behaviour itself may result in the touching or showing of the individual's or others' genitals. Be aware that this could occur as a means of avoiding a situation.
C: The person becomes sexually aroused as a consequence of another activity or experience, but without any sexual intent.

O'Brien's Five Accomplishments

O'Brien's Five Accomplishments (O'Brien, 1987) are essentially a checklist of what services should attempt to achieve for service users. They are:

- being present in the same place as ordinary citizens
- participating in the life of the community and making relation-ships
- making choices in all aspects of their life
- developing competence in all areas of life
- gaining respect from ordinary citizens.

Counselling and psychotherapy

Counselling skills offer another approach by which to clarify sexually motivated behaviours. The nature of the support that professionals working with people with a learning disability will find themselves providing may be to access resources, but more often, it will be to give their attention and actively to listen. This activity focuses on asking questions in a bid to gain a holistic picture of the client's needs and wishes, thereby enabling the person with a learning disability to make decisions and for the carer to offer appropriate information about how to move forward with their particular issues. The counselling provides a framework for a problem solving approach. Here the professional is not offering therapy and is not perceived as doing so. If however the person with a learning disability requires a counsellor/psychotherapist, then a suitably qualified practitioner can be sought.

Sexuality can be viewed as a learned behaviour (psychodynamic and behavioural theories). This is a useful approach when observing someone who is displaying sexual behaviour, as this may be an indicator of sexual abuse. Other theories (person-centred work and Gestalt) can, if appropriate, be integrated to offer a creative approach. The following excerpt from a case study illustrates this integrated approach in using counselling skills.

Case study

Sally is a young woman of 22. She lives with a small group of men and women who all have a learning disability. She has lived in this home setting for four years and enjoys a varied and full life. Prior to this she lived with her family, where she experienced physical, verbal and sexual abuse. It was during her transition from her family into her now established home that Sally accepted the opportunity of counselling sessions with a community nurse (LD) who also had training as a counsellor.

Diagnosed as having a moderate learning disability, Sally was able to communicate verbally and express herself well. She was however, less able to share her thoughts and feelings in relation to her family. This was not so much to do with her disability, but her confusion over her feelings towards her family and how they treated her. To enable Sally to gain confidence in sharing her thoughts and feelings, a creative approach was adopted. Initially the sessions focused on Sally and her nurse building a therapeutic relationship. Exercises were used that offered Sally the chance to draw whatever she felt was uppermost in her thoughts during a session, using a large sketch pad and felt tip pens. This gave Sally a framework in which she felt safe to draw and say a little to explain her pictures. It was she who was driving the work, not the nurse. This was a new and potentially risky experience for her, although progressing at Sally's pace enabled her to remain motivated and to stick with the process.

Later sessions focused on particular past incidents or aspirations for the future. Here the counsellor offered another creative structure, where Sally drew a picture of dreams that she wanted to make a reality (see Fig. 7.1). A similar exercise in Sunderland and Engelheart (1993) *Drawing Your Emotions* serves as a useful tool to enable individuals to express and understand their feelings. As with any experiential material it needs to be introduced and used sensitively and with care.

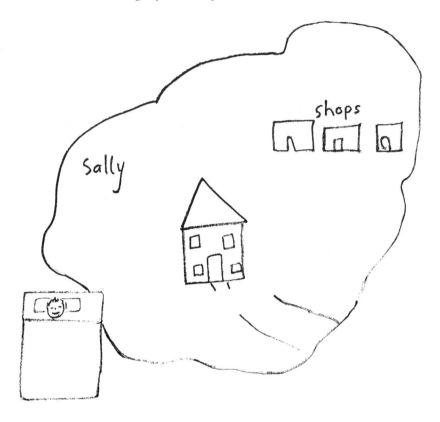

Fig. 7.1 My Best Dream.

Sally's dreams for the future are to further her education including literacy classes (hence her writing her name), and at some point to move into her own accommodation, where she would be near to the shops and could choose who came to see her at home.

Enabling Sally to take the lead during her sessions was not always successful. If her family had made contact with her during the preceding week, then the session was nurse led, as Sally expressed her wish for more structure, thereby relinquishing some of the control she had taken previously. This process of 'emotional holding' did not result in Sally becoming passive. Rather it helped her to manage the more painful parts of her life. This in turn resulted in her deciding to take back the control later in the same session or at the next session. She also chose to take a copy of her work home with her and used it as a vehicle to talk with her key worker about her particular care needs.

This particular case example reinforces some of Kennedy's (1996) findings in reviewing the research evidence on the myths surrounding abuse and children who have a learning disability. These are that children with a learning disability would be more likely to make false allegations and not benefit from therapeutic treatment. It is not that skill, talent or expertise has been missing. 'Rather, the lack has been around a reticence to allow creativity, flexibility, adaptability and innovatory ways of working with people with learning difficulties to occur naturally.' (Waitman & Reynolds, 1992, p.205)

Sexuality, commitment and marriage

The majority of people wish to have a long-term relationship with another person in their life. In today's society that may be fulfilled both within and outwith a marriage. In focusing on marriage part of the commitment will in many instances be to have a family. This commitment is still questioned as being appropriate for people with a learning disability, although reviews of marriages between this group have shown that with specific support around life skills and professional help, most do not experience greater problems than the population at large (Craft & Craft, 1979).

It is the tailoring of a multidisciplinary approach to meet the needs of a couple that is the key. Planning to enable psychosexual development through education and counselling in parallel with a life skills programme will offer the couple the opportunity to learn and to maintain their independence. This may go on to include fulfilling parenthood (Cross, 1994).

Sexual activity and risk

Sexual activity amongst people with a learning disability is more widely accepted than it used to be but brings with it the concerns that affect anyone who is sexually active. Sexually transmitted diseases including HIV infection demonstrate that sexuality can be risky and has the potential for working against those who are vulnerable, such as people with a learning disability. Brown (1992) views O'Brien's Five Accomplishments as the 'best framework we have to refer to in making judgments about how to address sexual and other service dilemmas ... applying these to HIV and sexuality issues shows that there are no easy answers'.

Leaving individual staff to take decisions involving risk tends not to happen, which reduces the opportunities for the person with a learning disability. There is a need for a well defined framework in which there is a process of sharing decisions. This does not avoid making decisions, rather it reduces the stress of taking sole responsibility for decisions by using a process of consensus.

The right of people with a learning disability to have a full life that includes employment, leisure and relationships brings with it the responsibilities of engaging in those activities. Focusing specifically on sexuality, a person with a learning disability may understand what it is to be sexually active; what needs to be established is whether or not they understand the consequences of their sexual behaviour.

Cambridge and Brown (1997) suggest a number of questions that professionals and carers can ask so that the appropriate responses are made in relation to 'people's understanding and appreciation of sex, safer sex and risk' (p.169). The questions are designed to ascertain whether or not the person with a learning disability understands that they are:

- at risk of HIV from sex
- able to reduce the risk of HIV and still have sex
- able to practise safe sex.

This begins to formulate a foundation on which to build more detail, thereby responding to risk management by asking how much knowledge or understanding the person with a learning disability has about sex, HIV and AIDS. This in turn offers a way forward to be formulated including providing education and advice.

Learning about personal relationships and sex

The issue of sexual vulnerability does not only relate to sexual abuse but also includes the issue of sexual safety and the need for sex education. The amount of literature relating to sex education programmes for people with a learning disability has increased over the last decade (Craft & Craft, 1983; Craft, 1994; Rushton, 1995). Formal evaluations of the impact of such programmes have also been undertaken (Craft, 1991; Lindsay *et al.*, 1994; Newens & McEwan, 1995).

People with a learning disability may, as has been highlighted by the Department of Health (1995) 'have difficulty using information and advice about contraception and safer sex... They are also less likely to receive peer messages about safer sex practices... [They] often have reduced opportunities for making long term relationships, and there is an increased incidence of abusive sexual experience.'

Using this statement as a foundation, the health programme to be provided needs to be delivered in a framework that is innovative and creative on the one hand and non-threatening and informal on the other. The following outline illustrates how six two-hour workshops for a personal relationships and sexuality programme could be run.

The workshops would focus on:

- personal relationships (including getting to know one another within the group and sharing feelings)
- personal relationships (who am I and how do I feel?)
- making and maintaining relationships (skills building)
- language (e.g. colloquialisms relating to relationships and sexuality)
- taking care of myself (positive body image and the resources available to help)
- sexuality (physical sexuality, safety and personal responsibility).

The workshops can be adapted for an adolescent or adult group setting. The exercises should be flexible so that they can be tailored to groups with a breadth of experience and a variety of abilities. The opportunity to learn and share together through a facilitative style will enable the participants to develop skills and confidence in responding appropriately to personal and sexual issues. Rushton (1995) ran a series of workshops specifically for adults with severe to moderate learning disabilities. A joint initiative between health and education service provision in Scunthorpe offered a similar programme for children with a learning disability, as part of their curriculum in a special school. This was a collaborative venture between the teaching staff, the school nurse and a nurse from the community team for learning disability.

Both these programmes were underpinned by the need for social and interpersonal skills development. This includes how the individual views things and how to relate to others, in terms of basic communication skills, e.g. eye contact, listening, attending. This is taken further by looking at how friendships and relationships are formed, maintained and the skills required to achieve this. Aspects of basic anatomy and health issues are dealt with within a positive framework 'well woman, well man' (Rushton, 1995, p.42). Issues around sexuality, thoughts, feelings and behaviours are then brought into focus. This includes the physical aspects of sexuality, safety and expectations.

Evaluations of sex education programmes have shown that myths have been dispelled and that the participants' assertiveness has increased as a result of taking part. There is a cautionary note that suggests that the participants may become overcompliant (people-pleasing behaviours) and that this could lead to possible exploitation. The following quote reflects the outcome to be achieved by any personal relationship and sexuality programme: 'You do not have to go out on a date and if someone kisses you it does not necessarily mean they love you' (Lindsay *et al.*, 1994, p.72). The point has been made by Newens and McEwan (1995) that it is most beneficial for the participants if groupwork is followed up by a series of one to one sessions for individuals. This comment is also borne out by McCarthy and Thompson (1992) who emphasise this approach for those who are already sexually active.

It is important to offer a flexible approach in delivering a programme of sex education by tailoring the content and method of learning to the group setting, together with input designed for individuals in a one to one setting. The drive to improve health both at local and national level is resulting in the development of programmes with the aim of reducing teenage pregnancies (DoH, 1998b). Although these are not specifically targeted at people with a learning disability, it would be an opportunity missed if this specific group of adolescents were excluded. More recently, picture books and leaflets have been produced as part of the NHS Cancer Screening Programmes (2000). These are to help women with learning disabilities understand breast and cervical screening, enable them to make a choice about accessing the service, and prepare them for the possible outcomes having undertaken the screening process. This drive is not only coming from a health perspective but also from a social one, designed to promote the independence of the individual.

Offering a sex education programme to people with a learning disability is only part of the picture. Parents, carers and professionals, also need to be educated. 'Nurses in all specialisms need adequate training if they are to deal sensitively with their clients' personal relationships' (Moore, 1991). This statement, while accurate, needs to go further. Nurses need to know how to go about incorporating psychosexual care as part of their practice. A personal perspective is valuable as part of coming to terms with our own sexuality, but this also needs to be further developed. It is still a part of human development that can cause acute embarrassment for the person, their parents or professionals involved with them. Enabling effective communication about sexual matters is not a matter of understanding just the mechanics of sexuality. It is the opportunity to develop a framework within which an open exchange of information between parents, professionals and the person with a learning disability can exist. For this to take place appropriately, adults need to be confident and relaxed about their own sexuality.

Conclusion

People with a learning disability are vulnerable, particularly when making or maintaining relationships. They may have a degree of physical sexual development, but be unable to choose or to consent to a sexual relationship. This seemingly negative statement goes against the philosophy of normalisation (Wolfensberger, 1972) and the rights of people with a learning disability. Perhaps the confusion arises from focusing on a full sexual relationship, rather than developing people's sexuality. Sexuality is not just a mechanical act. It is about communication, caring and loving. Those people with a severe and profound disability present the greatest challenge, as they are unable to give their consent and may be perceived to be restricted by the present legislation. How the development of a person's sexuality is managed without being defined as abusive is difficult and requires nurses, other professionals and parents to involve those with a moderate learning disability to formulate guidelines and policies. It is not acceptable for those of us involved in the care of people with a learning disability to ignore this part of their lives.

References

Belsky, J. (1980) Child maltreatment: an ecological integration. *American Psychologist*, **35**, 4, 320–35.

Brown, H. (1992) Sexual issues for people with learning difficulties. *Nursing Standard*, **7**, 12, 54–5.

Brown, H. & Barrett, S. (1994) Understanding and responding to difficult sexual behaviour. In: A. Craft (ed.) *Practice Issues in Sexuality and Learning Disability*. Routledge, London.

Cambridge, P. & Brown, H. (eds) (1997) *HIV and Learning Disability*. BILD publications, Plymouth.

Carr, L.J. (1995) Sexuality and people with a learning disability. *British Journal of Nursing*, **4**, 19, 1135–41.

Coxe, W. (1779) Annual register In: J. Ryan & F. Thomas (1986) *Politics in Mental Handicap*. Free Association Press, London.

Craft, A. (1991) Living your life programme. *British Journal of Special Education*, **18**, 4, 157–60.

Craft, A. (ed.) (1994) *Practice Issues in Sexuality and Learning Disability*. Routledge, London.

Craft, A. & Craft, M. (1979) *Handicapped Married Couples*. Routledge, London.

Craft, A. & Craft, M. (1983) *Sex Education and Counselling for Mentally Handicapped People*. Costello, London.

Cross, J. (1994) The right to choose. *Nursing Times*, **90**, 39, 60–62.

DoH (1995) *The Health of the Nation: A Strategy for People with Learning Disabilities*. Department of Health, London.

DoH (1998a) *Modernising Social Services*. Department of Health, London.

DoH (1998b) *The New NHS*. Department of Health, London.

Elwood, S. (1981) Sex and the mentally handicapped. *Bulletin of the British Psychological Society*, **34**, 169–71.

Fenwick, A. (1994) Sexual abuse in adults with learning disabilities. *British Journal of Learning Disabilities*, **22**, 53–6.

Garbarino, J. & Stocking, S.H. (1980) The social context of child maltreatment. In: J. Garbarino & S.H. Stocking (eds) *Protecting Children from Abuse and Neglect: developing and maintaining support systems for families*. Jossey Bass, San Francisco.

Gaze, H. (1992) Unspeakable acts. *Nursing Times*, **88**, 8, 14–15.

Kennedy, M. (1996) Sexual abuse and disabled children. In: J. Morris (ed.) *Encounters with Strangers: Feminism and Disability*. The Women's Press, London.

Koegel, P. & Whittemore, R.D. (1983) Sexuality in the ongoing lives of mildly retarded adults. In: A. Craft & M. Craft (eds) *Sex Education and Counselling for Mentally Handicapped People*, pp.213–40. Costello, London.

Lindsay, W.R., Michie, A.M., Staines, C., Bellshaw, E. & Culross, G. (1994) Client attitudes towards relationships: changes following a sex education programme. *British Journal of Learning Disability*, **22**, 70–73.

McCarthy, M. & Thompson, D. (1992) Teaching difficulties. *Community Care Inside*, 28 May, 2–3.

Moore, K. (1991) Confronting taboo. *Nursing Times*, **87**, 42, 46–7.

Morris, J. (ed.) (1996) *Encounters with Strangers: Feminism and Disability*. The Women's Press, London.

Morris, R.W. (1994) *Values in Sexuality Education*. University Press of America, Lanham, MD.

Newens, A.J. & McEwan, R. (1995) AIDS/HIV awareness training for young people with severe learning difficulties: an evaluation of two school programmes. *Journal of Advanced Nursing*, **22**, 267–75.

NHS Executive (1998) *The New NHS*. NHS Executive, London.

NHS Cancer Screening Programmes (2000) *Good Practice in Breast and Cervical Screening for Women with Learning Disabilities*. NHS Cancer Screening Programmes, Department of Health, London.

O'Brien, J. (1987) A guide to life-style planning: using the activities catalogue to integrate services and natural support systems. In: B. Wilcox & G.T. Bellamy (eds) *The Activities Catalogue: An alternative curriculum for youth and adults with severe disabilities*, p.175. Brookes, Baltimore.

Pearson, V. *et al.* (1998) Only one quarter of women with learning disability in Exeter have cervical screening. *British Medical Journal*, **316**, 7149.

Reid, D.A. (1995) Sexual activity in people with profound learning disabilities. *British Journal of Learning Disabilities*, **23**, 56–8.

Robinson, L. (1998) Screening women with learning disabilities. *Links*, **23**, 4.

Rushton, J. (1995) Learning capers. *Nursing Times*, **91**, 16, 42–3.

Ryan, J. & Thomas, F. (1986) *Politics of Mental Handicap*. Free Association Press, London.

Sobsey, D. (1994) Sexual abuse of individuals with intellectual disability. In: A. Craft (ed.) *Practice Issues in Sexuality and Learning Disability*, p.94. Routledge, London.

Sunderland, M. & Engelheart, P. (1993) *Drawing Your Emotions: creative ways to explore, express and understand important feelings*. Winslow Press, Bicester.

Taylor, G., Pearson, J. & Cook, H. (1998) Family planning for women with learning disabilities. *Nursing Times*, **94**, 40, 60–61.

Tredgold, A. (1908) *Mental Deficiency – Amentia*. Ballière Tindall, London.

Turk, V. & Brown, H. (1993) The sexual abuse of adults with learning disabilities: Results of a two-year incidence survey. *Mental Handicap Research*, **6**, 3, 193–216.

Waitman, A. & Conboy-Hill, S. (eds) (1992) *Psychotherapy and Mental Handicap*. Sage, London.

Waitman, A. & Reynolds, F. (1992) Demystifying traditional approaches to counselling and psychotherapy. In: A. Waitman & S. Conboy-Hill (eds) *Psychotherapy and Mental Handicap*. Sage, London.

Wilcox, B. & Bellamy, G.T. (eds) (1987) *The Activities Catalogue: An alternative curriculum for youth and adults with severe disabilities*. Brookes, Baltimore.

Wolfensberger, W. (1972) *The Principle of Normalisation in Human Services*. National Institute on Mental Retardation, Toronto.

World Health Organization Regional Office for Europe (1986) *Concepts for Sexual Health*. WHO, Copenhagen.

121

8. Sexuality, Fertility and Reproductive Health

Philippa Sully and Barbara Walters

Sexuality is integral to our personal identity as individuals and in society. We develop a sexual sense of ourselves through developmental processes, our interactions with others, life experiences and our individual differences (Bancroft, 1989). The purposes of human sexual behaviour (Bancroft, 1989) most relevant to this chapter are the promotion of bonding and intimacy between sexual partners, assertion of masculinity and femininity and the procreation of children. Bancroft also identifies expression of power as a function of human sexual behaviour, which seems important when looking at the ways in which health care relating to fertility and its control is delivered.

That emotional attachment is an essential part of human interaction is well documented (Bowlby, 1989; Murray Parkes *et al.*, 1991). It is arguable that how we grow and develop throughout life is influenced by the nature of our capacity to attach and maintain attachments (Erikson, 1963; Rutter, 1981; Bowlby, 1989; Murray Parkes *et al.*, 1991). In adulthood, one of the ways we demonstrate our development and status in the adult world is through the capacity to establish and maintain an exclusive sexual attachment to another adult, and possibly to demonstrate the success of our sexual attachment – and our identity and status as women and men (Pfeffer & Woollett, 1983) – through having children. Levinson (1986) and Roberts and Newton (1987) identify couple attachments and the establishment of a family (among other issues) as significant developmental stages that influence our sense of who we are as individuals and in society.

When exploring the impact of fertility on sexuality and its expression, it needs to be viewed in the wider contexts of the development of adult self-identity, relationships and social status.

122

Private and public domains: social expectations of women and men and childbearing

Cultural and social norms surrounding fertility, childbearing and rearing have a long history. Such a vital human function has rituals and expectations that are passed down through the generations and the centuries.

How we express our sexuality in public is carefully regulated. Rites of passage – engagement, marriage, birth and ceremonies that welcome the new infant such as circumcision and baptism – are the public face of the usually very private act of sexual intercourse. Babies are the public face of the sex act. However, certain demonstrations of sexual affection such as between lesbians and gay men, are not often acceptable in wider society.

To the authors, fertility and its control covers the span of avoiding pregnancy through abstinence or contraception, choosing to have an abortion, celebrating pregnancy and the arrival of a baby, to seeking help should individuals and their partners not succeed in achieving a pregnancy when they try to do so. This view is supported by Everett (1995). But social expectations concerning fertility and its control seem to focus largely on women and the choices they make to control their fertility (Shattuck & Schwarz, 1991). This is evident in the emphasis of contraceptive options being largely for female use, and reproductive technologies (although treating both male and female difficulties) focusing on the alteration and control of women's reproductive cycles (Shattuck & Schwarz, 1991).

Sandelowski (1986, p.446) argues that 'socialization makes motherhood the only real path to self-realization and normality for women'. That women's identity is an integral part of their status as mothers is evident in much of what they do – paid and unpaid – as adults (Crawshaw, 1995). When women in heterosexual relationships have difficulty conceiving, whatever the reason, not only is there a severe impact on their sense of power, choice and worth (Shattuck & Schwarz, 1991) and self-identity (Crawshaw, 1995), but also there is an implicit assumption that they are to blame, despite the fact that not all fertility problems are a result of female reproductive malfunctioning. This attitude of blame is evident in the medical terminology used to describe women's fertility difficulties 'incompetent cervix', 'hostile mucus' (Shattuck & Schwarz, 1991) as well as critical attitudes to women who have postponed childbearing in order to gain economic independence and fulfilment in paid employment.

The ability to establish an adult couple partnership, and possibly have children, is integral to women's and men's sense of who they are and their self-worth. Where people feel blamed or are blamed for their capacity to have or not to have children (witness highly publicised recent political debate in the United Kingdom on the 'irresponsibility' of single mothers) the emotional impact and consequent knock-on effect for a sense of self can be devastating (Sandelowski *et al.*, 1990).

The social norm is that it is expected that heterosexual couples will have children. It is common for women to be asked when having a termination of pregnancy 'Why don't you want this pregnancy?'. Likewise, when a baby has not appeared after what friends or family deem an appropriate time, they have been known to take it upon themselves to ask the couple when they intend to have children. The assumption is that they will have children. Common questions asked of childless couples are: 'When do you intend to start a family?'; 'Why don't you have any children?'. It also seems socially acceptable for individuals with children of their own to ask those who do not have children, or those pursuing fertility treatment, why they want a family.

Infertile couples have disclosed to the authors that they are then left with having to choose between explaining aspects of the most private parts of their lives or risk offending well-meaning but insensitive friends, family and professional practitioners. It is worth pondering on how commonly those who ask others about their plans for parental status, ever ask themselves 'Why did I want a baby?'.

Self-image, sexuality and fertility

In their study in the United States of 53 infertile couples and 10 fertile couples, Sandelowski *et al.* (1990, p.199) found that all the infertile couples entered their marriages with a 'presumption of fertility'. However, unlike the men in the study, not all the women, fertile and infertile, had taken their fertility for granted. When this aspect of their self-image was challenged, participants, particularly women, felt 'the entire self was damaged' (Sandelowski *et al.*, 1990, p.203).

Olshansky (1987) defines the entry into infertility treatment programmes as a 'formal identity' of being infertile. Prior to this individuals or couples assume an 'informal identity' as infertile, should they not have conceived as planned but also not sought treatment. Sandelowski *et al.* (1990) questioned this view, saying that the people in their study did not necessarily adopt a self-image of being infertile in order to deal with this aspect of their lives. Nonetheless, infertile couples, lesbians and gay men who seek to have children through assisted conception have to make public aspects of their most intimate lives to healthcare professionals.

How does an infertile person view her- or himself as a creative and fertile individual when the outside world views infertility as 'a terrible disease affecting our sexuality and wellbeing' (Winston, 1985, cited in Foster, 1995, p.49)? Sandelowski *et al.* (1990, p.199) found that infertile couples' distress was exacerbated by the fact that it was only when they chose to seek help with their infertility, i.e. to make a private aspect of their lives public, that their difficulty was transformed from 'an exclusively reproductive disease' entailing some obligations from society, to 'a reproductive choice entailing none'. Although society puts obligations on couples to have children and bring them up appropriately, infertile couples in this study found themselves without any sense that society offered them anything more than a marginal place in sociocultural ideas about disease.

That homosexual couples usually inhabit societies that expect they will not have children is largely self-evident and has been described as 'part of the deal'. Where does this leave the lesbian or gay couple who want children of their own? Are they too, to be subjected to the types of enquiries that heterosexual couples are less likely to encounter? It seems that society will accept that men's drive to have children is natural. However it is less willing to accept that women who are not in heterosexual relationships have a drive to become mothers (Foster, 1995). That motherhood is a relationship between mother and child, not necessarily dependent on whether or not the woman is in a heterosexual relationship (Pfeffer & Woollett, 1983, p.19), is an important concept to consider when looking at the impact of society's expectations of women and their roles. When women seek help to conceive, either as independent women without fertility problems, or because they have failed to conceive, it seems important that healthcare professionals are aware of the assumptions they may make about the lifestyles of those who are seeking their help with – i.e. making public – something that is essentially a very private matter.

Infertility is also seen as an affliction that befalls couples. Most of the research reviewed for this chapter was related to heterosexual couples, not individuals. The individual who is aware that she or he is infertile still has to deal with this onslaught on their self-identity. What do you say to a new sexual partner? Who else needs to know about this? If you plan to marry, does the rabbi need to know? Jews should 'Go forth into the world and multiply'. Is this grounds for the partner to break off any commitment to marriage? Suddenly a private matter becomes public.

Where the media learn of 'different' couples or individuals seeking to have children there have been vociferous expressions of moral outrage. Foster (1995, p.60) cites numerous examples of this, for example Ann Winterton MP described self-insemination as 'immoral and unnatural'. The implied statement here is that donor insemination carried out by a member of the medical profession in the treatment of an infertile heterosexual couple is acceptable. The feminist argument is that self-insemination 'strikes at the very heart of male control over women' (Foster, 1995, p.60). It can therefore be argued that, if Bancroft (1989) is correct, the control that the medical profession is allowed to maintain over women's and gay men's capacity to have children, is not only political, but sexual in nature.

There is a difference between the distress of infertility and the distress of infertility treatment. Solomon (1988) argues that in campaigning against reproductive technologies, feminists have not differentiated between these issues. This arguably leaves infertile feminists without the support of those women who share their view of women's experience. Here again the public discourse on a private matter leads to the social isolation of the infertile.

The explosion of reproductive technology has arguably led to the implication that couples who pursue treatment can be screened both emotionally and physically to produce 'better' children born to appropriately caring parents. In his study of counselling for clients seeking IVF treatment, Pengelly (1995, p.90) identifies that all the counsellors involved were concerned as to 'Whether it was part of their function to help assess a couple's suitablility to be offered treatment, for example in terms of their emotional stability and potential to care for a child.'

The experience of pregnancy, childbirth and adoption

Pregnancy, childbirth and adoption have rites of passage that recognise the position of new parents in their social world – the private becomes public. Where particular relationships have lower social standing – the lesbian or gay relationship, or that of the single mother with her child – these rites of passage can be minimised or excised. Consequently it is arguable that this transition to parenthood is more difficult for people without the support of public ritual and social recognition.

For many couples, the woman's pregnancy is an important part of proving that their bodies are functioning normally – men are fertile and women can do what women do. For men, not being fertile 'casts doubts on their masculinity, on their manhood' (Snowden & Snowden, 1984, p.15). For women, being pregnant proves their ability to conceive and have the special status of women (Houghton & Houghton, 1977).

Read (1999, p.588) describes pregnancy as 'a transition from one physical state to another . . . first pregnancy . . . a transition from one state of being to another'. As discussed above, the rites of passage related to major life transitions such as pregnancy are ways of recognising that these private events have huge personal and social implications. When at last people who have been infertile achieve a pregnancy it too has an impact on their sexual identity. Life will never be the same again, whether the pregnancy ends successfully or not.

How the individual and/or couple see themselves will be affected by their conscious and unconscious ideas about pregnancy, parenthood and the nature of sexuality in relation to these states. Read (1999) points out that where the pregnancy occurs after infertility or a history of miscarriage, fetal abnormality or neonatal death, there may be high levels of anxiety. These can be related to the physical experience of pregnancy or the emotional and social impact of this new state.

Pregnancy can also affect the couple's relationship where one or both might feel that the woman is increasingly unattractive with the advancing weeks. Myths surrounding the wisdom and effects of having sexual intercourse during pregnancy can influence couples' capacity for sexual intimacy. These, alongside physical ailments associated with pregnancy can in turn affect sexual expression and enjoyment. It is a tragic reality that many women experience violence and abuse from male partners when they become pregnant, thus underlining the vulnerability of women to male expressions of power in relation to sexuality.

The joy at finally achieving the longed-for pregnancy can be accompanied by ambivalence at the new social and emotional significance of impending parenthood and all that this entails. Sometimes when couples have invested a great deal of time and emotional, physical and financial effort into achieving a pregnancy this can become the pivot on which their relationship hinges. The longed-for pregnancy might then result in the relationship foundering, because one or both partners finds that there is little else left of the relationship outside this one shared aspect of their lives. But experiencing pregnancy and childbirth is only part of the process – parenting is something else again.

The transition to parenthood for infertile, expectant and new parents is a process which involves the 'added work of negotiating the ambiguity of infertility', redefining their fertility status and working hard to rebuild their sense of who they are in the world (Sandelowski, 1995). This process is one in which couples have to relinquish their identity as infertile and find a sense of themselves in society as parents.

How do couples or individuals feel when they are deprived of the human experience of creating a new life? Where they might adopt a child and become parents, they will have the experience of being parents, but they will still not experience creating a new life together. Adoption is therefore not a solution to infertility, although it is a solution to childlessness.

Emotional processes, sexuality and the finality of having no offspring

Throughout history infertility has caused deep sorrow to and rejection of individuals. Zaccharias and Elizabeth, the parents of John the Baptist, waited many years before conceiving a child. Sadly, childlessness is grounds for divorce in some societies and women can be put aside because they are barren, regardless of the cause.

Genetic death means that we leave no living aspect of ourselves behind. Coming to terms with this is identified in the literature (Hirsch & Hirsch, 1989, cite five sources) as a process of grieving. Letting go is integral to the resolution of grief. Sandelowski *et al.* (1989) in their study of 40 fertile and infertile couples (predominately white, middle income and in their 30s) describe a process of seeking a baby which they call 'mazing'. The process of 'reframing desire', choosing either treatment, adoption or to confront their infertility and remain childless, involved 'asking the right questions, confronting self, revelation and letting go' (Sandelowski *et al.*, 1989, p.225). It was extremely demanding of emotional, physical and financial resources, but couples weighed pros and cons of choices and tried to avoid decisions that would leave them with regrets. But this process only relates to those who have the means or desire to pursue parenthood publicly. Many others remain outside the public face of infertility treatment. What impact does this have on their self-esteem and their intimate and social relationships?

Successful pregnancy does not seem to improve previously

infertile women's emotional wellbeing (Bernstein *et al.*, 1988). Infertility reduces couples' sexual satisfaction – women being particularly vulnerable to this (Slade *et al.*, 1992) and some infertile people 'attach failure to conceive to their entire sexual identity' (Hirsch & Hirsch, 1989). It seems tragic that at a time of stress when nurture and intimacy are probably most needed, infertile couples find sexual expression less satisfactory.

Slade *et al.* (1992) in their three-year follow-up of infertile and fertile couples found that if couples remained infertile their anxiety, depression and hostility remained at levels identified at the beginning of the study. Infertile men had poorer self-esteem than those whose relationships were infertile for other reasons, and were more likely to use negative coping strategies than women who remained infertile. However, marital adjustment among the infertile couples remained good despite the impact that male infertility had on emotional, marital and sexual functioning.

Women seem more inclined, along with their male partners, to identify themselves as 'masculine' as they develop aspects of their lives which do not relate to childbearing and rearing (Hirsch & Hirsch, 1989). But they are more likely to feel general discontent than infertile men, possibly as a consequence of their sense of hopelessness and frustration as their longed-for child does not arrive. Men however, seem able to manage their infertile identity 'more successfully' (Hirsch & Hirsch, 1989, p.18).

This research seems to imply, by the way it is written and its findings, some value judgements about which aspects of women's and men's roles are desirable and acceptable. For example there is a suggestion that in comparison with men there is some sense that women are not as 'successful' as men in managing the distress caused by their infertility. The literature reviewed here identifies explicitly and implicitly the impact social expectations about sexual behaviour and fertility have on individuals' sense of themselves, their sexual identity and their sense of well-being.

It seems significant that most of the research into the impact of infertility on people focuses on couples rather than individuals. A high profile is given to the more technological or spectacular sorts of fertility treatment and care for homosexual couples is rarely if ever discussed. Lesbians seem to have been be excluded from the right to IVF treatment, as in theory are single women, according to current UK legislation governing reproductive techniques (Doyal, 1995). How much these implied and explicit values wound and isolate the infertile or those who choose parenting styles outside the norm, can only be speculated upon.

Feminist perspectives and the control of fertility

Morse (1995) identifies four essential components when teaching women's health from a feminist perspective. They are *diversity, dominion, equity* and *merit*. When looking at the context and extent of fertility control from contraception through to abortion and assisted conception, it seems that these principles apply equally well to the delivery of these services. Health professionals who apply these principles will offer creative and sensitive care to the women and men who seek help for such personal aspects of their lives.

That we all automatically make assumptions about the nature of sexuality and lifestyles is only human. To use those assumptions to exert power or sustain prejudice is, the authors suggest, ethically questionable. The feminist principle that the personal is the political is clearly evident in the way in which contraceptive, abortion and assisted conception services are offered – individual professional practice is informed and sustained by the society in which it takes place. That professional practitioners in these fields have a responsibility to those in their care to question the assumptions they make about who is worthy of care, why and how they will deliver that care, seems self-evident.

In the delivery of high quality care or medical insurance to support that care, the authors are of the view that it is essential to value each person as unique and different and to celebrate the diversity of human nature and experience. Infertile people feel powerless, without choice, and even blamed for their lot. By allowing choice and autonomy in fertility control methods or infertility treatment options (Reading *et al.*, 1989, cited in Slade *et al.*, 1992), professional practitioners and members of the interdisciplinary team can help vulnerable people to exercise a sense of dominion over their bodies and lives at a time when they often feel vulnerable and that they have little or no power.

Women and men – regardless of their state of fertility, sexual preferences and marital status – are, the authors believe, entitled to equal treatment. Likewise, people are worthy of the best fertility care on offer because they merit this as people, despite prevailing sexual and cultural norms.

Shattuck and Schwarz (1991) describe a nursing model which spans medical models and the social context and psychological needs of clients which could go some way to understanding the parameters of infertile people's experiences, as well as developing care processes that are sensitive to individuals' needs within the macro- and microcontexts in which care is delivered. This model could be equally well applied to contraceptive and abortion services.

The authors are of the view that it is not possible to remove fertility control from the public arena. There is too much at stake, from diminishing world resources exacerbated by rapid population growth and inequity in consumption and wealth distribution, to shattered self-esteem and sense of purpose as a result of infertility and the consequent disruption of couples' (and, the authors suggest, individuals') taken-for-granted worlds (Williams, 1984, p.197, cited in Sandelowski *et al.*, 1990). Nonetheless, sexual intimacy is largely expressed privately. In seeking help to avoid or achieve a family, individuals and couples offer professional practitioners the awesome privilege of allowing them into perhaps the most private aspect of their lives.

References

Bancroft, J. (1989) *Human Sexuality and its Problems* (second edition). Churchill Livingstone, Edinburgh.

Bernstein, J., Mattox, J.H. & Kellner, R. (1988) Psychological status of previously infertile couples after a successful pregnancy. *Journal of Obstetrics, Gynaecological and Neonatal Nursing*, November/December, 404–8.

Bowlby, J. (1989) *A Secure Base*. Penguin, Harmondsworth.

Crawshaw, M. (1995) Women-centred counselling in reproductive medicine. In: S.E. Jennings (ed.) *Infertility Counselling*. Blackwell Science, Oxford.

Doyal, L. (1995) Infertility counselling and IVF: the moral and legal background. In: S.E. Jennings (ed.) *Infertility Counselling*. Blackwell Science, Oxford.

Erikson, E. (1963) *The Child, The Family and the Outside World*. Penguin, Harmondsworth.

Everett, H. (1995) Termination and limitation: a social worker's perspective. In: S.E. Jennings (ed.) *Infertility Counselling*. Blackwell Science, Oxford.

Foster, P. (1995) *Women and the Health Care Industry*. Open University Press, Buckingham.

Hirsch, A.M. & Hirsch, S. (1989) The effect of infertility on marriage and self-concept. *Journal of Obstetrics, Gynaecological and Neonatal Nursing*, January/February, 12–20.

Houghton, P. & Houghton, D. (1977) *Unfocused Grief: Responses to Childlessness*. The Birmingham Settlement, Birmingham.

Levinson, D.J. (1986) A conception of adult development. *American Psychologist*, **41**, 1, 3–13.

Morse, G.G. (1995) Re-framing women's health in nursing education: a feminist approach. *Nursing Outlook*, **43**, 6, 273–7.

Murray Parkes, C., Stevenson-Hinde, J. & Marris, P. (1991) *Attachment Across the Life Cycle*. Routledge, London.

Olshansky, E.F. (1987) Identity of self as infertile: An example of theory generating research. *Advances in Nursing Science*, **9**, 54–63.

Pengelly, P. (1995) Working with partners: counselling the couple and collaborating in the team. In: S.E. Jennings (ed.) *Infertility Counselling*. Blackwell Science, Oxford.

Pfeffer, N. & Woollett, A. (1983) *The Experience of Infertility*. Virago, London.

Read, J. (1999) Sexual problems associated with infertility, pregnancy, and ageing. ABC of sexual health. *British Medical Journal*, **318**, 7183, 587–9.

Roberts, P. & Newton, P. M. (1987) Levinsonian studies of women's adult development. *Psychology and Aging*, **2**, 2, 154–63.

Rutter, M. (1981) *Maternal Deprivation Reassessed*. Penguin, London.

Sandelowski, M. (1986) *Sophie's Choice*: a metaphor for infertility. *Health Care for Women International*, **7**, 439–53.

Sandelowski, M. (1995) A theory of the transition to parenthood of infertile couples. *Research in Nursing and Health*, **18**, 123–32.

Sandelowski, M., Harris, B.G. & Holditch-Davis, D. (1989) Mazing: infertile couples and the quest for a child. *Image: Journal of Nursing Scholarship*, **21**, 4, 220–26.

Sandelowski, M., Holditch-Davis, D. & Harris, B. (1990) Living the life: explanations of infertility. *Sociology of Health and Illness*, **12**, 2, 195–215.

Shattuck, J.C. & Schwarz, K.K. (1991) Walking the line between feminism and infertility: implications for nursing, medicine, and patient care. *Health Care for Women International*, **12**, 331–9.

Slade, P., Raval, H., Buck, P. & Lieberman, B.E. (1992) A 3-year follow-up of emotional, marital and sexual functioning in couples who were infertile. *Journal of Reproductive and Infant Psychology*, **10**, 233–43.

Snowden, R. & Snowden, E. (1984) *The Gift of a Child*. George Allen & Unwin, London.

Solomon, A. (1988) Integrating infertility crisis counselling into feminist practice. *Reproductive and Genetic Engineering*, **1**, 1, 41–9.

Williams, G. (1984) The genesis of chronic illness: narrative reconstruction. *Sociology of Health and Illness*, **6**, 175–200. Cited in M. Sandelowski *et al.* (1990) Living the life: explanations of infertility. *Sociology of Health and Illness*, **12**, 2, 195–215.

Winston, R. (1985) Why we need to experiment. *The Observer*, 10 February. Cited in P. Foster (1995) *Women and the Health Care Industry*. Open University Press, Buckingham.

9. *Sexuality and Later Life*

Hazel Heath

On the journey through life, older age is not the destination but a period of experience. Each person makes his or her unique journey and, as with all aspects of life, how we express sexuality, enjoy relationships or experience intimacy runs as a thread through our individual development. As we each approach older age, our attitudes will have been influenced by the prevailing values and norms during our formative years as well as our experiences of sexual expression and relationships. Generalisations, particularly related to later life, have little predictive value for individuals, but the weight of research and anecdotal evidence clearly indicates that the majority of people want to continue to have the option to express themselves as sexual beings and to enjoy their chosen relationships throughout their lives.

Two pervasive inhibitors of older people's sexuality in contemporary western society are the myth that sexual interest is inappropriate to feel and the stereotype that its expression is unwelcome. Although arguably society is gradually changing its view, older people may remain caught up in the negative and discouraging attitudes which surround sexuality in later life, as a quote from an interview in Thompson *et al.* (1991) illustrates:

> 'Ben is very aware that an older man's sexuality is widely disapproved of. He risks being scorned as "a dirty old man". He argues that this is the wrong view. "There's no difference – older people doing what younger people do – you've got the same ingredients to make it". But then he cannot admit to his family that he has these longings. "There's something wrong with me – there must be – I shouldn't be thinking about women at my age".'

This chapter analyses the construction of sexuality in later life and some key influencing factors. It identifies relevant literature and the

133

limitations within this. It explores some positive aspects of relationships in later life, alongside problems that may arise. It concludes with suggestions on how the concept of sexuality might be reframed in older age and examples of how older people, and nurses who work with them, can help to overcome problems towards more fulfilling expression of sexuality throughout later life.

The construction of sexuality in later life

An individual person's sexual self-image and self-identity are constructed through a number of influences – the images and cultural norms which surround us, perceptions of our current situations and experiences on which we draw.

Societal attitudes, expectations, prevailing images and cultural norms

Western society generally promotes the message that sexuality and sexual need decline in later life. Many of the images portray stereotypes of older people as either 'false teeth and stair lifts' or 'deliriously fit and enjoying a marvellous sex life' (Matthews, 1999). In a youth orientated culture, the strong underlying message is that, in order to maintain sexual attractiveness, the ageing process must be avoided or suppressed (Pointon, 1997). Sex is perceived as natural for young and even for middle aged people, but not for older people. Men who continue to express sexual interest into older age may be portrayed as 'dirty' or 'lecherous'; women who continue to dress stylishly into older age may be described as 'mutton dressed as lamb' (Gibson, 1992a). In this way, society imposes 'age' identities – i.e. sexual interest should cease at a certain age and older people should dress more sombrely. This can have a very negative effect on an older person's ability to view life positively, particularly in the field of sexual expression (Littler, 1997).

Self-image is also linked to ideas of value or usefulness to society. If the prevailing culture removes the opportunity for older people to contribute and feel useful, this can profoundly affect self-identity, and society effectively controls older people in this manner. This is known as social age-control theory (Littler, 1997). In current older generations the usefulness of men in particular to society may have been experienced through work. Compulsory retirement removes the opportunity for this. Women's social usefulness may be linked to reproduction and family rearing. When women have gone through the menopause and their children have left home, self-identity may be similarly affected. However, the social construction

134

of self-image is arguably distinct between the genders. Desirable attributes in males, such as competence and autonomy, can be maintained into later life. Older men are not uncommonly described as handsome or distinguished. Desirable attributes in females tend to be around youth and beauty. Older women are rarely described as beautiful.

Negative social attitudes may be reinforced by younger family members. This is particularly so for an older parent who obtains a new partner. Even adult children with permissive attitudes about sexual behaviour among their contemporaries may be unable to accept that their father or mother wishes to engage in sexual activity, more so when the partner is not the other parent (Pointon, 1997). There may be many reasons for this such as resentment of a new partner taking the place of a parent or concerns about loss of inheritance, but these attitudes can have constraining effects on older people, as is illustrated in the appendix of Butler and Lewis (1988)

> 'Children will sometimes try to preserve the memory of their deceased parent ... you can then find yourself accused by being selfish, insensitive or disloyal; and if they succeed in making you feel guilty, you may be compelled to sever your new relationship. This is a mistake.'

Gibson (1992b) goes further in claiming that young people have a vested interest in 'castrating' older people – life is more convenient for them if older people are docile and sexless.

The influences of the norms of a particular subculture can also influence the social construction of sexual self-identity, for example in the case of homosexuals and lesbians (Quam & Whitford, 1992). Older homosexual men experience similar problems to those of ageing people generally (Pointon, 1997), but being identified as 'old' within the social group may occur earlier in gay communities, even as young as 40. Community identity can be particularly important for gay men and, if younger men dominate the public gay community, older gay men can feel rejected or even repressed (Langley, 1997).

Generational influences, moral values or religious doctrines

Fundamental values influence decisions about what is right or wrong, appropriate or inappropriate to think, feel or do, and ultimately 'should I or shouldn't I?'.

People's values and means of sexuality expression are influenced by the values and norms of behaviour promoted in their formative years, as well as their experiences through life as it unfolds. Chapter 2 describes how the permissive and rebellious attitudes of 1960s teenagers was nurtured by the views of motherhood prevailing in the early 1950s. Those currently old were possibly influenced by the Victorian morality of their parents, for example that sex was primarily for procreation within marriage and masturbation was a self-violation. People who have never had the opportunity to talk openly about sex will likely find it difficult to do so in later life. Greengross and Greengross (1989, p.34) describe how

'women who grew up before the Second World War generally expected little pleasure from sex.... Few wives expected their husbands to satisfy their sexual needs and often experienced a sense of deep guilt and anxiety that they might be abnormal even to have such feelings.'

Legislation also influences values and behaviour and, for older people, penetrative sex between two males has been illegal in the UK for most of their lives. Older people may possibly therefore exhibit more restrictive attitudes to same sex relationships than younger people because of the attitudes prevailing during their formative years. Deevey (1990) suggests that older gay men and lesbian women may be especially secretive because of family rejection in their younger years, religious condemnation, legal or medical discrimination or even homophobic violence.

Body image and age-related changes

Physical age-related change can affect how individuals feel about themselves as sexual beings and about being valuable, attractive or desirable. They can also impact on sexual functioning and, particularly if the individuals are not aware of the normal changes which occur with ageing, can lead to much anxiety and frustration as well as ultimately a cessation of sexual activity.

In order to become aroused, both men and women often require more direct, intensive and prolonged genital stimulation than they did at a younger age. This can be difficult to seek from partners, particularly if discussing sex is not the norm in the relationship. Older women often experience vaginal dryness due to oestrogen depletion. They may find orgasm takes longer to achieve and orgasmic sensation is reduced. Older men usually find that their erections become less firm and the angle of erection changes from 45 to 90 degrees. They may find that they are unable to ejaculate on some occasions and sensation may be reduced when they do ejaculate. The refractory (recovery) period between erections can be prolonged. If individuals are aware of these changes, they can more easily come to terms with them and adopt different lovemaking practices (Riley, 1994).

Many of the pathological causes of change in sexual functioning can occur at any age but those particularly common in later life include the following (Riley, 1999).

Debilitating disease

Some people give up sexual activity because of the cumulative effects of chronic illness (see Chapter 14); due to fear of another attack after an acute episode, such as a myocardial infarction or stroke (see Chapter 13); or as a consequence of the experience of diagnosis and treatment, for example Shell and Smith (1994) describe how physical and emotional changes caused by diagnosis and treatment of cancer are often compounded in the older patient. Endocrine abnormalities, not uncommon in later life, can reduce sex drive in both sexes and cause a range of complications.

Pain

This may be local, e.g. coital pain due to vaginal dryness or loss of elasticity of the vagina and related structures (which can be reversed by hormone replacement therapy) or in other areas of the body, such as osteoporotic back pain or arthritic hip. Arthritic hip may also prevent hip abduction and commonly used positions for intercourse (see Chapters 14 and 16).

Drugs

Many frequently prescribed drugs are known to reduce or impair sexual function and reduce sexual drive (see Chapter 16).

Many of these problems can be remedied through sensitive and appropriate counselling, education and treatment. Riley (1999) reports that erectile function can now be restored in a large proportion of older men provided they are not too embarrassed to seek help and the doctor does not feel it inappropriate to treat an elderly man.

Psychological adjustment and coping

Changes occur throughout life but those in later life are particularly unwelcome when they are associated with loss. Greengross and Greengross (1989, p.35) write that older people 'are often deeply affected by a string of losses: the loss of their job as they approach retirement age, of their children as they leave home, of their own parents as they die or become frail and dependent and very often the irreparable loss of their [husband/ wife/partner] if they are widowed.'

Most people, and particularly those in the current older generations, adapt to change and continue with life. However, the cumulative effects should not be underestimated, as the following quote from a 76-year old man responding to a survey (in Brecher, 1984) demonstrates:

'I've been widowed, alone, for eight years, so my sex life is zero – nothing. My wife was sick nine years, so there have been 17 years of inactivity. I'm sure I'm useless for there hasn't been an erection for years ... being old ... and ugly is a terrible combination – so I keep myself busy in my yard... But I do miss a woman very much... Being lonely and old is just as bad as being lonely and young – and I've known both... No love, not even anyone to touch, or hold their hand.'

Literature on sexuality in later life

Research

Research into desires, needs, sexual activity and relationships among older people is fraught with methodological problems. Some research ignores the older population altogether, thus reinforcing the common stereotype. A recent large scale survey in Britain was much vaunted as comprehensive (Wellings *et al.*, 1994), but the upper age limit of the sample was 59.

There are other problems such as the following.

- Most research originates in the USA and is not therefore wholly applicable to UK culture.
- There is virtually no literature which acknowledges the ethnic or cultural diversity of the UK.
- Even studies which do acknowledge older people may contain very small samples. In Kinsey *et al.*'s classic studies (1948, 1953), only 185 of a total sample of 12,000 in the first study were over 60, and his conclusion that 75% of 80 year olds are impotent was based on a sample of four people. Similarly, although Masters and Johnson's laboratory studies were hailed as a breakthrough in understanding of the role of ageing in sexual functioning, they

included only 31 individuals aged over 60 out of a total of 694 (Gibson, 1992a).

- Sample bias is also common. For example, despite older women constituting the greater proportion of older people, White (1982) found that older men are more frequently studied. There is also a bias in some studies, where the samples skew towards a white, middle class, male and heterosexual perspective (Jackson, 1996) and non-institutionalised older people (e.g. Starr & Weiner, 1981; Bretschneider & McCoy 1988).
- Many studies use cross-sectional, rather than longitudinal, methodologies (i.e. they sample different cohorts from different age groups rather than following one cohort as they age). Cross-sectional studies commonly make no allowance for generational or cohort effects. George and Weiler (1981) recorded the sexual activity of older people with a partner over six years and found that the generational effect was greater than the effect of ageing. Kellett (1993) emphasises that the age-linked decline in sexual activity suggested by cross-sectional studies is 'much greater than that which is found in practice' (p.310).

Most research concludes that a decline in sexual activity, or the ability to enjoy it, are not inevitable consequences of ageing. The most recent large-scale study to include older people, conducted in the USA, concluded that people over the age of 65 'do not want to be relegated to the rocking chair and are often as sexually driven as they were in their youth' (Janus & Janus, 1993, p.28). 'The greying segment of Americans may be leading the way to superior sexual experience' (p.22).

Books for and by older people

Since the early 1990s a number of books have been written about sexuality in later life to highlight issues around ageing and relationships (for example Greengross and Greengross, 1989; Gibson, 1992a, b; Gibson, 1997; Sherman, 1999). Some are written by older people for older people, or feature the experiences of older people.

Clinical literature

The volume of clinical literature focusing on sexuality and older people has gradually increased over recent years. The range now covers clinical literature, mainly written by specialists in psycho-sexual medicine; gerontological papers, written by specialists in various gerontological fields; and a range of nursing literature from both the USA and the UK. For a fuller review see Heath (1999a). One area where there is virtually no literature is sexuality in older people from minority ethnic groups. At the time of writing, the number of older people from ethnic minorities is small, but this will soon begin to increase markedly, and it behoves nurses to learn about the range of people with whom they will be working and to be open and sensitive to their individual needs. Situations may arise where, for example, a woman's cultural norms prescribe that she does not undress in the presence of men and is only able to show her body to her husband or women from her own sect. Misunderstandings will be compounded if the person is not able to communicate easily, or does not speak English and there is no one to interpret.

Relationships in later life

Establishing, maintaining, changing or ending relationships can be complex at any time in life but there are distinct aspects in later life and among the current generations of older people.

Long-term partnerships

People in current older generations tended to marry for life. Many describe how they overcame early problems and became closer to their partner in later life.

> 'Those of us fortunate in having long-lasting and successful marriages will have outgrown the need to impress or to try to change the other, having now learnt tolerance in the areas where we differ. A distinct advantage as we get older is to have someone with whom we can be totally honest. This can help us in accepting ourselves more easily as the people we are, rather than those we used to have hopes of becoming. A close relationship with our partner is for many of us the foundation stone on which we build the last part of our lives.'
>
> (Greengross & Greengross, 1989, p.12)

Some describe how intimacy and lovemaking became enhanced later in life.

> 'Now that the children are grown and gone, we are delighted to be a single couple again ... we find that our shared experiences have made us closer, wiser and funnier ... we like being able to make love in the afternoon if we wish, or to wait a few days

longer than usual if one or another of us is not in the mood. It's a lovely time of life.'

(Brecher, 1984, cited in Gibson, 1997 p.129)

However, there can be particular difficulties in lifelong partner- ships. Partners can become bored, can experience different needs or levels of sexual desire, or to cease to find their partner attractive particularly if they have changed markedly over the years or experience illness or disability. Even lifelong partnerships can experience difficulties if regular sexual contact is interrupted through acute illness or temporary absence of one partner, for example through hospitalisation. Riley (1999) reports that, in such circumstances, it is not uncommon for couples to experience diffi- culty restarting sexual contact.

Loss of a partner

The greater one's age, the greater the likelihood of losing a partner. The death of a partner may remove one aspect of a person's identity as a partner or wife or husband as well as the immediate oppor- tunities for closeness and intimacy.

Constraints on relationships in later life may be demographic in that there are more older women than men, particularly in the very old age groups. There are currently around three times as many widows as widowers, and women over the age of 60 may find it difficult to find a new partner (Johnson, 1996) and commonly become companions. Open physical affection between women tends to be more socially accepted than between two men (Raphael & Robertson, 1980).

Developing new relationships

Developing new relationships can be daunting in later life, parti- cularly in the context of negative societal attitudes towards older people and sex. Nevertheless, new and fulfilling relationships are formed:

'I am a widow of 76. I lost my husband two years ago. At first I was devastated and, in spite of the wonderful support from my family, I could not really contemplate continuing my life. I was encouraged by an old and distant friend to find a voluntary job and make a new life for myself. I am now very much in love with the friend concerned. At my great age I did not recognise what was happening at first, but am now delighted to be so alive and happy. The world is warm and welcoming and so newly

141

beautiful. I would never have thought it possible to feel so happy and vital at my age.'

(Vera, from Gibson 1997, p.199)

Living alone and celibacy

Some people in the older generations have chosen to spend their lives without a partner, for example those whose loved one was killed in wartime, or for other reasons. Webb (1994) highlights that, because studies discussing 'single' women often make no distinction between those who have never married, those separated, divorced or widowed, little is known about the health of never-married, nulliparous women.

Reframing sex in later life

The expression of sexuality in later life, and indeed the desire for such expression, are totally individual. Many factors influence each person's views, desires and needs and Riley (1999) suggests that these include:

- the degree of sexual activity in earlier life
- the enjoyment and fulfilment derived from sexual activity in previous experience
- individual feelings about age-related changes in physical appearance and sexual response
- feelings about seeking sexual activity in later life
- feelings of embarrassment or guilt about aspects which society generally might not condone, such as masturbating, using erotic stimuli or the services of professional sex workers
- particular difficulties in later life, e.g. monotony in a relationship, unresolved grief, seeking new partners, uncertainties about sexual performance.

Life changes, and particularly losses, can take their toll on a person's self-esteem and sexual self-concept. Gibson (1992a) believes that most older people may take some time fully to realise the physiological and psychosocial changes that will take place over the last 30 years of their lives and suggests that, if they hope to recapture precisely the same sort of sexual satisfactions that they had in youth and middle age, they will be disappointed. One factor which maintains sexual desire is sensual satisfaction. This includes not only sexual excitement, orgasmic sensation and physical relief from sexual tension, but satisfaction from pleasing the partner.

Riley (1999) suggests that this positive feedback in older partner-ships is not always forthcoming. If older men and women find it more difficult to become sexually aroused, sex may not be as satisfying as it was in their younger years.

Gibson (1992a) suggests a rethinking of the definition of sexuality for later life to change the emphasis away from phallic performance and orgasm towards pleasure, satisfaction, psychological content-ment, a sense of self-worth and a celebration of their love for their partner. He believes that if these are the real goals of lovemaking, rather than the more limited view, then people can successfully continue to enjoy sex well into old age. There are many ways to enjoy intimacy, physical stimulation, sexual expression and sexual pleasuring with or without intercourse. Riley (1999) confirms that many older people who remain sexually active are motivated primarily by the need to satisfy the need for intimacy, to feel needed and valued by, and connected to, their partner. At a time in life which can easily become dominated by feelings of loss, meaningful relationships, intimacy and sexual sharing can be a powerful affirmation of attractiveness and of self-identity – feeling wanted, desired, valued and enjoyed.

There are also physiological benefits of sexual activity in later life, which include the general benefits of enjoyable and meaningful activity; the benefits of cardiovascular and general physical exer-cise, increased blood flow to specific areas of the body (Kellett, 1989, 1993, 1996; Seymour, 1990) (for example orgasms in older women can help increase muscle tone within the pelvis and perineum and reduce urinary incontinence; see Drench & Losee, 1996; Roe & May, 1999).

Working with older people

Sexuality can be a highly challenging issue for nurses to address with any client but there are particular issues for nurses and older people. Working across generations can present challenges. Taken to an extreme, nurses and other carers may be up to four genera-tions younger than a patient. The formative influences on their perspectives on sexual expression will be very different.

Difficulties can also arise when nurses identify older patients with their parents or grandparents, a process known as counter-transference. As one nursing home nurse in Heath's (1994) inter-views remarked: 'The residents are the same age as my grand-mother – I didn't like to think of my parents having sex, let alone my grandparents'. If nurses are unsure of what to acknowledge regarding older people's sexuality, the assessment may produce care plans with comments such as 'not applicable', 'likes her hair set', or 'likes to be called Dorothy'. Research has demonstrated that, when practitioners are uncomfortable with their own sexuality and intimacy needs, they are at best blind to their older clients' sexuality, and at worst judgemental (Altschuler & Katz, 1996).

Framework for practice

The following ideas are offered as a basis for working with older people:

- *Individual persons:* try to understand older people as individuals – their values, desires, needs and hopes for the future.
- *Biographies and relationships:* try to view them in the context of their lives and their life journeys. Learn from them about their significant experiences and relationships. This is known as the biographical approach (for further reading see Schofield, 1994; Wells, 1998; Heath, 1999b).
- *Sexuality cues:* try to be sensitive, open and receptive to cues about their desires, choices or needs to express sexuality, in all its potential modes of expression (including personal presentation, roles in life, intimacy, relationships).
- *Knowledge, skills and experiences:* try to be aware of your own knowledge and areas of comfort/discomfort. Aim to enhance your understanding of how normal ageing affects individuals (biologically, psychologically, socially etc.) and how illness and disability can impact upon this.
- *Environment and 'permission':* try to create an environment which 'gives permission' for individuals to feel comfortable in raising issues of concern. Readers are referred to Chapter 16, which contains full discussion of levels of practice and intervention in terms of giving Permission, offering Limited Information, Specific Suggestions and Intensive Therapy (the P-LI-SS-IT model) (see Chapter 16).

Practice examples

By way of illustration, this chapter offers two examples of working with older people – those with dementia and those with, or at risk of, sexually transmitted infections.

Dementia

How older people with dementia who express sexuality are viewed and treated illustrates the stereotyping of older people generally as

144

asexual, the lack of understanding of people with mental health needs and the feelings of inadequacy experienced by nurses when trying to deal with sexuality expression. At least 75% of people over the age of 85 do not have dementia, but the incidence rises sharply with age. There is a great deal of misunderstanding and a dearth of research on sexuality and people with dementia and what literature there is clearly demonstrates that, in care settings, sexuality expression is viewed as being a 'problem'. Archibald (1998) found that the most common types of sexual expression reported by managers among nursing home residents with dementia were holding hands (male and female), male residents fondling breasts of female staff, male residents publicly and privately masturbating and male residents without dementia having a sexual relationship with female residents with dementia. In all of these situations, it is likely that the 'problem' arose in the staff, rather than the residents, because staff felt they ought to 'deal with things' but felt unsure how best to do this. Archibald's (1994b) flow chart can be helpful in identifying where both the problem and the solutions might lie (see Fig. 9.1).

Pritchard and Dewing (2001, p.21) emphasise that

> 'it helps to try to look at a person's behaviour as communication from someone who may feel ill and frustrated, who may be finding it difficult to express themselves and their needs, and who may be faced with a lack of understanding from those around them'.

A particular issue for people with dementia and those who work with them is loss of short-term memory: the person may forget that they have recently had sex. They may misrecognise another person and this is particularly understandable when a female carer is undertaking intimate care in a homely situation for a male resident who may have visual or hearing impairment.

Dementia can also result in sexual disinhibition and, for example, a person with latent homosexual desires may for the first time openly seek someone of the same sex, or someone who has experienced few or no partners may actively seek partners and obtain pleasure from the interactions. It is vitally important to recognise that the person with dementia is an adult being with adult status and possibly sexual needs. Adult status, which includes the acceptance of the person as a sexual being, is symbolised by autonomy, self-determination and choice (Archibald 1997, 1998). For further discussion, see Alexopoulos (1994); Archibald (1994a, b, c, 1997, 1998); and Haddad and Benbow (1993a, b).

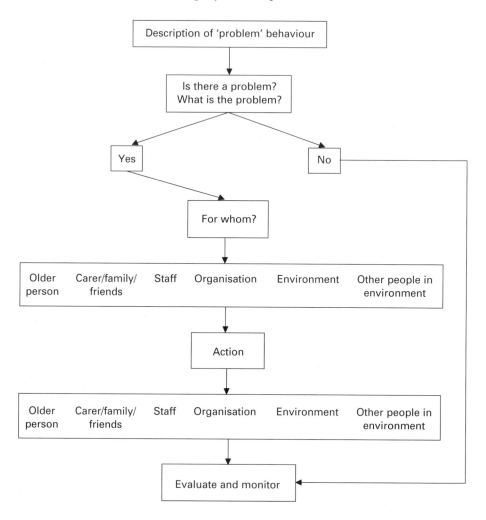

Fig. 9.1 Framework for action when the expression of sexuality is seen as a 'problem'. Adapted from Archibald, C. (1994b) Sex: is it a problem? *Journal of Dementia Care*, **2**, 4, 16–18.

The wishes, feelings and needs of partners must also be considered. They have probably experienced profound change in their relationship with the person with dementia, for example reciprocity may no longer be possible, considerable role change may have taken place as the partner becomes personal carer, or the person may seek sexual intimacy which the partner is no longer able to offer.

Sexually transmitted infections (STIs)

Working with older people with, or at risk of, STIs illustrates the impact of negative societal stereotypes, how generational attitudes can affect health behaviour, age-related changes and the distinct presentation of illness in later life, as well as the challenges of intergenerational working, and how older people themselves can take a lead in promoting health.

The stereotype of older people as asexual may actually result in them not receiving appropriate care. Doctors may not tend to consider HIV as a diagnosis in older people (Whipple & Scura, 1996) and nurses may not always take universal precautions with older people because they do not think of them as a risk group (MacGregor, 1994).

Although the research on STIs and older people is sparse, it is clear that they are as at risk as younger people, in some cases more so (Rogstadt & Bignell, 1991). They may not use a condom because there is no need for contraception. In women, diminished vaginal secretions and friable vaginal mucosa reduce protection from infection (Whipple & Scura, 1996). An increasing number of people over the age of 50 are being diagnosed as HIV positive or as having Acquired Immune Deficiency Syndrome (AIDS) (Marshall, 1997). The number of HIV cases in the over 50s rose by 94.5% from 1985–96, compared with a 10.4% rise in the total population, and the number of AIDS cases reported in the over 50 age group is larger than in the 24 and under age group (Public Health Laboratory Services AIDS Centre PHLS, cited in Marshall, 1997).

AIDS may not be readily recognised in older people because it tends to manifest differently and HIV-related illnesses tend to be more aggressive (Kendig & Adler, 1990). Symptoms such as fatigue, weakness, anorexia and weight loss may be assumed to be signs of ageing and may be difficult to diagnose, particularly AIDS-related dementia (Whipple & Scura, 1996). For many older people with AIDS, neurological symptoms are the first they will have. Pneumocystis carinii pneumonia (PCP) has been mistaken for chronic obstructive pulmonary disease or congestive cardiac failure. Bacterial infections, skin problems and respiratory complications may well be regarded as a normal process of ageing but could well be HIV-related disease (Grigg, 2000).

Gonorrhoea, if untreated, can cause a type of arthritis and inflammation of the reproductive organs, resulting in pelvic inflammatory disease or inflammation of the prostate or testicles. Despite the fact that arthritis and prostate problems are very common among older people, they are rarely linked to STIs. Some units for older people with mental health needs (EMU units) test for syphilis rather than HIV, but the incidence of syphilis is falling and that of HIV is rising (Grigg, 2000). Complications of severe STIs and particularly HIV can be greater for older people – weakness can lead to postural instability causing falls, tiredness causing pressure area risk, oral thrush can severely compromise nutrition, diarrhoea can lead to dehydration and further complicate skin breakdown.

Gott (1999) used a self-administered questionnaire, which was completed by 121 symptomatic older attenders at clinics in Leicester, Nottingham and Sheffield. Nearly 45% of them waited more than two weeks between seeing symptoms and coming to the clinic, preferring to 'wait and see'. Some of these said they were too embarrassed or afraid to attend. Older patients were over five times more likely to delay if they had had an HIV test in the past or intended to have one during their clinic appointment. These delays are significantly longer than those seen in younger patients. Gott (1999) concluded that older people are less informed about the need to have sexually transmitted infections treated as early as possible, as compared with younger patients.

Older people may not receive health promotion messages as these have primarily been directed at younger people. In addition, partly because of the 'countertransference' referred to above, nurses can find it difficult to do so. As Grigg (2000, p.17) suggests: 'Consider discussing condoms with an older patient and teaching him/her how to use one. How comfortable would you feel? Where would you advise them to obtain condoms or further advice?' Older people have clearly stated that they do want to know more about HIV and AIDS and educational material is now available (Age Concern, 1993). The Beth Johnson Foundation Publication *Healthy Sex Forever* (1996) was written for older people by older people who reported that they found it helpful to have the facts about healthy sex, not only for themselves, but in order to share the information with their grandchildren and younger people.

Conclusion

Sexual identity, sexual need and the desire for intimacy can continue throughout life but, as this chapter has illustrated, older people can be discouraged by ageist myths, societal stereotypes and the attitudes of those around them. The chapter has explored a range of issues distinct to later life. It has offered suggestions on how the concept of sexuality might be reframed and on how nurses and others can work with older people. Nurses can have a pivotal role in helping older people, particularly those with illness or disability, to express themselves in the way in which they would choose. By being open to a person's concerns, creating opportunities for him or her to talk and learning to become comfortable talking about sexual issues, nurses can help people articulate problems and deal with them.

It is important that nurses have the necessary knowledge and skills to be able to care for patients in this sensitive aspect of life and to work with them in a constructive and non-judgemental way (Grigg, 1997). The role of the professional is to help older people to realise their true feelings, and to work towards the creation of an environment that is conducive to the continuity of sexuality expression for those for whom it has constituted an important part of their lives.

References

Age Concern (1993) *HIV? AIDS? We're older gay men, it's not our problem.* Age Concern, London.

Alexopoulos, P. (1994) Management of sexually disinhibited behaviour by a dementia patient. *Australian Journal on Ageing*, **13**, 3, 119.

Altschuler, J. & Katz, A.D. (1996) Sexual secrets of older women: countertransference in clinical practice. *Journal of Clinical Gerontology*, **17**, 51–67.

Archibald, C. (1994a) Sex, drugs and prejudice. *Journal of Dementia Care*, **2**, 3, 20–21.

Archibald, C. (1994b) Sex: is it a problem? *Journal of Dementia Care*, **2**, 4, 16–18.

Archibald, C. (1994c) Never too late to fall in love. *Journal of Dementia Care*, **2**, 5, 20–21.

Archibald, C. (1994d) *Sexuality and Dementia.* University of Stirling, Stirling.

Archibald, C. (1997) Sexuality and dementia. In: M. Marshall (ed.) *State of the Art in Dementia Care.* Centre for Policy on Ageing, London.

Archibald, C. (1998) Sexuality, dementia and residential care: managers' report and response. *Health and Social Care in the Community*, **6**, 2, 95–101.

Beth Johnson Foundation (1996) *Healthy Sex Forever.* Beth Johnson Foundation, Stoke on Trent.

Brecher, E.M. (1984) *Love, Sex and Ageing.* Little Brown, Boston.

Bretschneider, J.G. & McCoy, N.L. (1988) Sexual interest and behaviour in healthy 80–102 year olds. *Archives of Sexual Behaviour*, **17**, 2, 109–29.

Butler, R.N. & Lewis, M.I. (1988) *Love and Sex after 60.* Harper and Row, London.

Deevey, S. (1990) Older lesbian women: an invisible minority. *Journal of Gerontological Nursing*, **16**, 5, 35–7.

Drench, M.E. & Losee, R.H. (1996) Sexuality and sexual capacities in elderly people. *Rehabilitation Nursing*, **21**, 3, 118–23.

George, L.K. & Weiler, S.J. (1981) Sexuality in middle and later life. *Archives of General Psychiatry*, **38**, 919–23.

Gibson, H.B. (Tony) (1992a) *The Emotional and Sexual Lives of Older People: A Manual for Professionals*. Chapman & Hall, London.

Gibson, H.B. (1997) *Love in Later Life*. Peter Owen Publishers, London.

Gibson, T. (1992b) *Love, Sex and Power in Later Life: A Libertarian Perspective*. Freedom Press, London.

Gott, C.M. (1999) Delay in symptom presentation among a sample of older GUM clinic attenders. *International Journal of STD and AIDS*, **10**, 1, 43–6.

Greengross, W. & Greengross, S. (1989) *Living, Loving and Ageing: Sexual and Personal Relationships in Later Life*. Age Concern, London.

Grigg, E. (1997) Guidelines for teaching about sexuality. *Nurse Education Today*, **17**, 1, 62–6.

Grigg, E. (2000) Sexually transmitted infections and older people. *Elderly Care*, **21**, 1, 15–19.

Haddad, P. & Benbow, S. (1993a) Sexual problems associated with dementia: part 1, problems and their consequences. *International Journal of Geriatric Psychiatry*, **8**, 547–51.

Haddad, P. & Benbow, S. (1993b) Sexual problems associated with dementia: part 2, aetiology, assessment and treatment. *International Journal of Geriatric Psychiatry*, **8**, 631–7.

Heath, H. (1994) Sexuality in later life: How nurses in continuing care environments facilitate the expression of sexuality in older residents. Unpublished, MSc Thesis, University of Surrey, Guildford.

Heath, H. (1999a) *Sexuality in Old Age*. Nursing Times Clinical Monographs No 40. Emap, London.

Heath, H. (1999b) Perspectives on ageing and older people. In: H. Heath & I. Schofield (eds) *Healthy Ageing: Nursing Older People*. C V Mosby, London.

Jackson, S. (1996) Heterosexuality and feminist theory. In: D. Richardson (ed.) *Theorising Heterosexuality*, pp.21–38. Open University Press, Buckingham.

Janus, S. & Janus, C. (1993) *The Janus Report on Sexual Behaviour*. John Wiley, London.

Johnson, B.K. (1996) Older adults and sexuality: a multidimensional perspective. *Journal of Gerontological Nursing*, **22**, 2, 6–15.

Kellett, J. (1989) The reality of sexual behaviour in old age: there's a lot of it about. *Geriatric Medicine*, **19**, 10, 17–19.

Kellett, J. (1993) Sexuality in later life. *Reviews in Clinical Gerontology*, **3**, 309–14.

Kellett, J.M. (1996) Sex and the elderly male. *Sexual and Marital Therapy*, **11**, 3, 281–8.

Kendig, N. & Adler, W. (1990) The implications of AIDS for gerontology research and geriatric medicine. *Journal of Gerontology*, **45**, 3, 77–81.

Kinsey, A.C., Pomeray, W.B., Martin, C.E. & Gehard, P.H. (1948) *Sexual Behaviour in the Human Male*. WB Saunders, Philadelphia.

Kinsey, A.C., Pomeray, W.B., Martin, C.E. & Gephard, P.H. (1953) *Sexual Behaviour in the Human Female*. WB Saunders, Philadelphia.

Langley, J. (1997) *Meeting the Needs of Older Lesbians and Gay Men*. (Report 97/2) Health and Social Policy Research Centre, University of Brighton, Brighton.

Littler, G. (1997) Social age cohort control: a theory. *Generations Review*, **7**, 11–12.

MacGregor, H. (1994) Risk exposure. *Nursing Times*, **90**, 47, 55–8.

Marshall, T. (1997) Infected and affected: HIV, AIDS and the older adult. *Generations Review*, **7**, 4, 9–11.

Matthews, V. (1999) An age apart from the consumer. *Financial Times*, 5 November.

Opaneye, A.A. (1991) Sexuality and sexually transmitted diseases in older men attending the genito-urinary clinic in Birmingham. *Journal of the Royal Society of Health*, **111**, 1, 6–7.

Pinfold, S.M. (1994) The joys of ageing. *Care of the Elderly*, April 1994, 140–44.

Pointon, S. (1997) Myths and negative attitudes about sexuality in older people. *Generations Review*, **7**, 4, 6–8.

Pritchard, E. & Dewing, J. (2001) Someone else's problem? Older people with dementia in acute settings. *Nursing Older People*, **12**, 10, 21–6.

Public Health Laboratory Service AIDS Centre, Communicable Disease Surveillance Centre and Scottish Centre for Infection and Environmental Health. Unpublished Quarterly. Cited in T. Marshall (1997) Infected and affected: HIV, AIDS and the older adult. *Generations Review*, **7**, 4, 9–11.

Quam, J.K. & Whitford, G.S. (1992) Adaptation and age-related expectations of older gay and lesbian adults. *Gerontologist*, **32**, 3, 367.

Raphael, S. & Robertson, M. (1980) Lesbian and gay men in later life. *Generations Review*, **6**, 16.

Riley, A. (1994) Ageing and the physiology of sex. *Care of the Elderly*, March 1994, 92–6.

Riley, A. (1999) Sex in old age: continuing pleasure or inevitable decline? *Geriatric Medicine*, **29**, 3, 25–8.

Roe, B. & May, C. (1999) Incontinence and sexuality: findings from a qualitative perspective. *Journal of Advanced Nursing*, **30**, 3, 573–9.

Rogstad, K. & Bignell, C. (1991) Age is no bar to sexually acquired infection. *Age and Ageing*, **20**, 377–8.

Schofield, I. (1994) A historical approach to care. *Elderly Care*, **6**, 6, 14–15.

Seymour, J. (1990) Sexuality in the elderly. *Care of the Elderly*, **2**, 315–16.

Shell, J.A. & Smith, C.K. (1994) Sexuality and the older person with cancer. *Oncology Nursing Forum*, **21**, 3, 553–8.

Sherman, B. (1999) *Sex, Intimacy and Aged Care*. Jessica Kingsley, London.

Starr, B. & Weiner, M. (1981) *The Starr–Weiner Report on Sex and Sexuality in the Mature Years*. McGrath, New York.

Thompson, P., Itzin, C. & Abendstern, M. (1991) *I Don't Feel Old*. Oxford University Press, Oxford.

Victor, C. (1987) *Old Age in Modern Society*. Chapman & Hall, London.

Webb, C. (1994) Never-married women's health in old age. In: C. Webb (ed.) *Living Sexuality: Issues for Nursing and Health*. Scutari Press, London.

Wellings, K., Field, J., Johnson, A.M. & Wadsworth, J. (1994) *Sexual Behaviour in Britain. The national survey of sexual attitudes and lifestyles*. Penguin Books, Harmondsworth.

Wells, D. (1998) Biographical work with older people. In: E. Barnes, P. Griffiths, J. Ord & D. Wells (eds). *Face to Face with Distress: the professional use of self in psychosocial care*. Butterworth Heinemann, Oxford.

Whipple, B. & Scura, K. (1996) HIV in older adults. *American Journal of Nursing*, **96**, 2, 23–8.

White, C. (1982) Sexual interest, attitudes, knowledge and sexual history in relation to sexual behaviour in the institutionalised aged. *Archives of Sexual Behaviour*, **11**, 1, 11–21.

10. *Sexuality and People who are Dying*

Elizabeth Searle

Two of the subjects that cause most apprehension in nursing are sexuality and death/dying, yet unless we are able to explore the relationships between both, we risk offering inadequate care to people who face death. Caring for people who are dying is still an area riddled with inequalities. These particularly exist between the specialist palliative care services extensively supplemented by major charities, which champion the need for people to prepare for death, to accept death and to celebrate life until death, compared with the care that acute and non-specialist services are able to offer. Yet even in specialist palliative care services, sexuality is not always addressed as openly as it might be and there is little literature about sexuality and dying to guide our practice.

This chapter attempts to address the complex area of sexuality in people who are dying and to explore what it might mean to them. Searching for a broad and useful definition of sexuality, the chapter offers an adapted *Theory of Love* alongside a *Model of Loss*. It acknowledges the culture and context within which much palliative care takes place and the constraints and boundaries which influence expression of sexuality. The chapter does not seek to give answers to all of the challenges but to raise awareness, provoke thinking about practice and, most importantly, to promote a realisation that there is still much to do in this area of care.

The context of palliative care

The culture and context within which most palliative care has historically taken place exerts the single most significant influence on the provision of holistic care. The steady increase in palliative care services was born of the visions of individuals such as Douglas

Macmillan, founder of Macmillan Cancer Relief, Dame Cecily Saunders of St Christopher's Hospice and the Marie Curie organisation, who championed the care of dying people as a holistic process involving spiritual, social and psychological aspects, as well as the physical. Much as these services have considerably enhanced the care offered to dying people and their families, the voluntary funding source and Christian values have created a context that can control or limit the expression of sexuality. It may present difficulties for patients and partners discussing sexual issues with nurses – perhaps akin to 'talking sex with angels', and particularly so if their partnerships or sexual activity would be condemned in Christian teaching. This was highlighted at the height of the moral media backlash against HIV and AIDS when, concerned about fund-raising revenue, hospices refused to offer palliative care services even to those suffering from Kaposi's sarcoma. This position was unchallenged by Dame Cecily Saunders (1986). The far-reaching effects of the need to control the expression of sexuality are demonstrated through the calls received by a gay bereavement project. Callers had been refused health care. Same-sex partners failed to obtain legal recognition, which led to the loss of shared homes following death. The medical profession had refused to accept same-sex partners as next of kin so they were unable to obtain information on a gay partner's health. The church refused gay people the sacrament and partners felt compelled to hide their relationships at funeral services (Cave, 1993).

Palliative care is now well recognised as a speciality in nursing and medicine, rightly so in the eyes of many who argue that this can only benefit patients by concentrating skills, knowledge and research. Nevertheless, there remains a danger that a paradigm shift could occur away from viewing death holistically as a psychosocial experience towards a more biomedical focus, the so-called medicalisation of the dying (James & Field, 1992; Biswas, 1993). The skilful assessment and treatment of complicated symptoms should not detract from a holistic approach with open communication about death and dying and within which issues of sexuality can be explored.

In addition, people die in a range of settings, many not within specialist palliative care. Largely determined by sources of funding, palliative care services have tended to focus on the care of people with cancer, and patients in palliative care settings do not always reflect the cultural mix of the local population (Rees, 1997). While specialist services are increasingly becoming available to patients with other diseases, particularly HIV/AIDS and some neurological conditions, many of the major causes of death such as vascular or coronary heart disease, are not readily linked with specialist palliative care services.

Whether access to specialist care will increase the opportunities for the sexuality of dying people and their partners to be addressed is open to question. However, regardless of setting, the culture of the service, the knowledge of staff and the training available will influence the courage and skills of practitioners to tackle difficult issues.

Images of sexuality and death

Images of sex and death influence our social construct and these have changed through history from the taboo and mystique of the Victorian era, the experimentation of the 1960s, and the 'sex equals death' hysteria promoted by the media post-HIV and AIDS (see Chapters 1–3).

Over centuries death and sex have been revealed in renowned works, such as those of William Shakespeare and John Donne. In such works death often results from suicide. The passion of forbidden love, and hence sex, found in *Romeo and Juliet* which leads to the well known ending may lead us to conclude that life without passionate love is so desolate that death can be the only release. At a time when both sex and suicide were forms of social and religious taboo, critics suggested that John Donne used sex and death as interchangeable concepts – as extremes of both excitement and fear.

Current media coverage of sex and death is similarly ambivalent. The messages are powerful and often subliminal. A survey of tabloid newspaper coverage of sex and death over a three-month period (Pickering *et al.*, 1997) revealed a range of skewed images. Death was frequently reported, but predominantly sudden untimely death. Other distortions included the pictures that accompanied the stories. For example, the death of Marlene Dietrich, who died in her 90s, was illustrated by pictures of her in her youth at her height as a sex symbol. A high percentage of time was dedicated to the death of young women where a sexual motive was suspected or mutilation occurred. The time and space dedicated to this outweighed the reality and the frequency of such crimes. The subsequent reporting of the reactions of the dead women's partners suggested a move from traditional male stoicism to one of emotional wreck and turmoil.

A powerful example of how societal images influence personal perspectives was the 'sex equals death' media message surrounding

HIV and AIDS in the early 1980s (see Chapter 3). In addition, the uncaring 'you only have yourself to blame' attitudes towards some groups in society were fuelled by the press because at that stage most people had little personal experience of HIV to moderate their views (Davenport-Hines, 1990).

When we consider sexuality and sexual behaviour we do so within the context of our personal experience and beliefs, informed by our upbringing and the influential messages to which we have been exposed. If asked to imagine a pair of lovers, our first image is most likely to be young, slim, fit, attractive and healthy people. We are unlikely to immediately picture a couple where one partner is old, disabled, frail, ill or near to death, where a great deal of manipulation and positioning of contorted, deformed bodies occurs before sex can take place. It is important that healthcare professionals do not allow media sensationalism to remove sex and death from the agenda of what is personally acceptable to contemplate, discuss openly and deal with constructively.

Sexuality and the end of life

People who are dying, even where there are no obvious signs, are generally sexually disenfranchised (Siemens & Brandzel, 1982). For sick people there are a number of expected ways to behave, summarised as the 'sick role' (Gorden, 1966), and the boundaries between patients and their professional carers are clearly defined. Being 'sick' excuses the person from normal sexual activity and in both acute and chronic illness both the patient and healthcare professional can freely accept this asexual state without challenge (see Chapters 13 and 14).

In acute healthcare settings, the traditional preparation of nurses focused on ill health needs and getting patients home quickly so that they could resume their normal lives. A comfort zone therefore existed for both patient and carer where sexuality need not be addressed. However, not every patient returns to his/her previous health state and indeed some die, with a need to live as complete and normal a life as possible for the time remaining. In order to achieve this, they will need healthcare staff to adopt non-judgemental attitudes, to redefine boundaries, to search out the knowledge and skills necessary for them to meet their needs and to face the challenges – to do the unthinkable – to discuss sex with the dying.

The literature on terminally ill patients and sexuality is very limited and much only explores the reasons for the problems.

Among the literature, the work of Wasow (1977) is noteworthy. During this study terminally ill patients showed a strong need to talk about their sexual needs and to continue their sexual relations. The benefit of sexual satisfaction and intimacy outweighed the pain, discomfort and drain on energy. Even in the face of distressing symptoms, the effects of altered body image, disfiguring surgery, wounds, and the fear of worsening disease which can occur towards the end of life, sexual needs clearly remain an important issue for people. To feel loved, to belong, to share the most intimate of experience with the one most important to them can help people to leave this world feeling that they may be missed but more importantly that they made an impression.

Defining unmet needs in people who are dying is not straight-forward. It depends on open and honest communication between the professional and the patient and the patient and his or her partner. It is also dependent on the acknowledgement of the partner whether that is someone of the same gender or an extra-marital relationship. It can be difficult to acknowledge complexities in the lives of others, for example working with guilt feelings that arise in a woman who has participated in extra-marital relationships, when her partner is dying. Or initiating a conversation around the topic of sexuality with a dying man who has met all his sexual needs, for many years, outside his marriage. Such situations can raise moral and ethical issues for practice if we consider facilitating this need but nevertheless these issues need to be addressed. In addition, it is important to acknowledge that the lack of a partner does not equate to a lack in sexuality.

A Model of Love and Loss

Sexuality is defined and expressed in many ways but can broadly be linked to the giving and receiving of love. In order to acknowledge the psychological and emotional processes in someone experiencing loss, I have mapped Sternberg's Theory of Love (1986) alongside Stedeford's Model of Loss (1994). While the strengths and weaknesses of both theories are important to reflect upon they are used here primarily as a framework within which to place the discussion.

Sternberg's theory suggests that there are three main components – passion, intimacy and commitment. These same three components can be applied to sexuality. For the relationship to be satisfying, Sternberg would argue that there should be a close match between our own and our partner's triangle when placed together. However each of the three components completing the triangle is defined uniquely by individuals – what passion means to you and how you like it demonstrated is individual, but you have a need for your partner to match your own interpretation and therefore meet your needs. Conversely partners need you to match their interpretation in order to meet their needs.

Unless each component is demonstrated by one to the other by being translated into action it is impossible for us to match it against our own needs and thus feel satisfied. This may account for the often used phrase 'I know he loves me, I just wish he would show it.' To follow this to its ultimate conclusion, for healthcare professionals to help dying patients and their partners they need to clearly assess what each component means for each patient and help their partner meet these needs.

In order to achieve this it is important to consider the feeling of loss that both partners will be experiencing on the diagnosis and prognosis of an incurable disease which will lead to the death of one. Stedeford's (1994) work on facing death is useful to consider here and, although used here merely as a framework, is worthy of further consideration.

Mapping these two models allows us to explore specific difficulties in meeting sexual needs and to suggest strategies for helpful advice or interventions.

Passion

The demonstration of passion from one partner to another may take many forms; touching, kissing, cuddling and requests for sexual activity and intercourse itself. Through these actions a clear message is given from one partner to another. However preoccupation with other emotional work will inevitably reduce the ability to demonstrate or need passion. For example on the diagnosis of an illness the shock and numbness identified by Stedeford will clearly reduce the overall need for the full demonstration of passion but may enhance the need for commitment and intimacy – a need to be reassured that the relationship is solid and will not falter. This timing may coincide with an admission to hospital where asexual status may be enforced.

It is vital that, on return home, as normal a relationship as possible is established. This can only occur if clear information is given to the couple regarding resuming sexual activity, such as the effects of certain medications or practical advice on physical limitations. However the shock and numbness felt by both partners are part of a process of anticipated loss (Worden, 1991) that may resolve with time.

Stedeford suggests that a period of psychological denial then occurs: 'it can't be happening' or 'it can't be me', but she argues that you can only deny something you are part way to believing. This denial, however, causes a period of buffering when normality continues while a slower acceptance can occur. It would be reasonable to assume that where the demonstration of passion has resumed it would continue here as if all is 'normal'. There is a need to hold onto 'normality' for as long as possible resuming, where able, all activities. Failure at this time could lead to a heightened experience of loss – a compounded and enhanced realisation that all is not well. The increased stress will of course impact on sexual expression and may result in erection problems for men and dryness or dyspareunia for women.

Anxiety is often a self-fulfilling prophecy in that 'fear of failure produces failure' (Hyde, 1994). The importance of support and understanding from the healthcare practitioner is vital, particularly explanation of the difficulties, encouragement to explore the areas of passion that are possible and practical advice, such as on lubricants etc. Where symptom control issues exist, advice can be given on how the partner may help. For example, massage can help reduce the sensation of pain by blocking pain impulses and creating a feeling of wellbeing; it can also be a demonstration of touch and tenderness. The use of essential oils where acceptable, particularly lavender or camomile to aid relaxation, can also compensate for odours that wounds and fungating tumours may produce. This helps promote touch where it was once feared or unpleasant. Clearly for satisfying sexual activity to occur the mind has to pay attention to the now and not be preoccupied with the 'maybes': open discussion will allow the may bes to be explored.

The demonstration of passion can continue to its fullest up until the very last days of life. Feeling wanted and desirable may well be a relief from feelings of grief and depression. It is important to acknowledge and communicate to partners that one of the best therapies at this time is the one only they can give. The demonstration of passion needs privacy and security. Patients spending large amounts of time in a hospital or hospice setting have a right to this basic requirement. Many institutions are now considering internal locks on the doors of side rooms with 'do not disturb' signs. Many hospices have double beds for side rooms. Yet there is much to do, particularly in acute care settings. Healthcare professionals can create an environment of acceptance and non-judgemental attitudes by recognising that patients have sexual needs and acknowledging the role that partners have to play.

Intimacy

The demonstration of intimacy takes the form of private and personal communications of feelings, personal information, emotional support and empathy. One can clearly see how sharing intimacy with a partner can facilitate the acceptance of loss. The role for the professional may be in supporting the partner to support the patient.

Research on intimacy is limited, but inventory tools such as Personal Assessment of Intimacy in Relationships (PAIR) (Schafer & Olson, 1981) uses indicators such as:

> My partner listens to me.
> My partner understands my hurts and joys.

Feelings of closeness and trust are important to intimacy yet consider the effects on these feelings within the common scenario when the partner is told the diagnosis before the patient. Not only does this prevent the patient from beginning a normal and natural grief process but also it immediately puts up barriers between the couple that reduces the ability to demonstrate intimacy and hence love. Fear of disclosing too much is a heavy burden for a partner to bear, particularly if the relationship is close. Within less open relationships this can encourage collusion and withdrawal at a time when encouraging closeness would be preferable. I suspect little thought is paid to the impact on sexuality in this undesirable situation.

For the surviving partner, moving through a grief process in anticipation of the loss may also necessitate withdrawal of emotional support. This is a form of coping – a kind of damage limitation – but detachment too early in the dying trajectory leaves the patient with unmet needs. It is a challenge for the professional involved to support this withdrawal while explaining this experience to the couple. Through redefining boundaries, the professional can form a trusting and therapeutic relationship and may be able to substitute the listening and emotional support needs of the patient, thus allowing a natural process of anticipated loss (Worden, 1991) for both to be supported.

Other stages identified by Stedeford, such as anger, clearly impact on the demonstration of intimacy. We are often only angry with the people who truly understand us, because it is a safe environment. We can be angry because they will understand – but do they? Professionals explaining anger as a natural emotion and part of a grief process can facilitate understanding, help the relationship to stay intact and thus allow intimacy to continue.

Commitment

Sternberg's third component is commitment, described as 'accepting the good with the bad', 'seeing it through' and 'being with' someone whatever the situation may bring. As health professionals know, the 'being with' often presents the greatest challenge. Watching a loved one die must be one of the most difficult experiences in life. Clearly no one could question the commitment of partners who stay throughout this situation, yet what choice do they have? Would society be tolerant of someone who decided enough was enough? When we think about it logically, of course we could not blame them for leaving, yet comments such as 'they don't visit every day' or 'they hardly talk to each other' are made with negative connotations. Supporting partners to maintain and demonstrate their commitment is a vital role for the professional and finding respite care or daytime relief may help. As the illness progresses, sleeping in a spare room or downstairs may seem easier, yet sleeping together can facilitate loving experiences that could not otherwise happen. Promote the moving of the double bed, does it matter if the room is cramped or bigger sheets need washing? Helping partners to be with their dying loved one is a major role for healthcare professionals.

Supporting strategies

From discussion of Sternberg's Theory of Love and Stedeford's Model of Loss, three main themes for consideration have emerged.

- The importance of facilitating the needs of the patient in areas of intimacy, passion and commitment.
- The importance of supporting the partner through communication and understanding to enable them to continue to demonstrate their love.
- The importance of acknowledging that patients without partners still have needs for intimacy, passion and commitment.

Symptom control and psychological approaches

Many of the physical changes experienced by people who are dying, and the treatments to minimise these unwanted effects, impact on the expression of sexuality and sexual activity. Clearly the symptoms themselves may cause difficulties, and good symptom control is paramount, but the combination of drugs often required to control symptoms will have a large impact on the meeting of sexual needs. Interestingly in many books about symptom control, information about the specific side effects of drugs do not extend to much more than morphine and constipation, almost as if side effects are considered irrelevant if one is dying. This apparent lack of information may lead us to speculate on the potential effects of medication on sexuality and I would encourage professionals to observe and learn through their experience. The following are offered as examples.

- Many of the drugs used for pain relief result in constipation, which can cause listlessness, nausea and discomfort with vaginal intercourse, but even more so with anal intercourse.
- Opiates can severely depress sexual behaviour and erectile dysfunction may be common. Explanation of this possible side effect is vital to couples particularly if normal relations are to continue or to resume as soon as possible.
- Side effects are not always negative, for example in the short term, morphine may increase sexual desire as a result of freedom from pain and a feeling of wellbeing – in this situation a window of opportunity exists for couples to affirm their relationship.
- Anti-cholinergic drugs used for drying secretions and occasionally nausea may cause erectile dysfunction as they inhibit the parasympathetic nervous system.
- Sedatives used to induce sleep may also suppress desire and sexual response but tranquillisers and antidepressants may enhance sexual response by improving the patient's mental state and sense of wellbeing.

Psychological aspects are equally important. People in pain, or those who are nauseated, fatigued and coping with death or loss may not be able to fulfil or require a sexually active role. Yet, as has been described, the need for love and the expression and receiving of love can be among the greatest experiences in life. They can offer an expression of passion, intimacy and commitment that can surpass that within specific sex acts. It is also never too late to learn. Even in relationships where love has not always been obvious, encouraging the demonstration of commitment may be helpful in facilitating grief for the remaining partner. Ambiguous and angry relationships are a risk factor for complicated grief reactions (Worden, 1991).

Practical considerations

Fear of increasing symptoms, and even making the illness worse, can restrict patients from experimenting with more comfortable sexual positions that are not claustrophobic and include no undue increase in pressure and weight. Perhaps more upright positions, or sitting or standing may help. Simple measures like emptying bowels and bladder, not eating for a couple of hours before and timing sexual activity to coincide with the peak of analgesic action or just simply at the best time of day are also helpful (see Chapter 16).

The use of syringe drivers for subcutaneous administration of medicines is now fairly common but the needle siting positions are not always ideal. Abdominal siting will cause problems for couples who wish to continue sexual activity or just to have a cuddle. Upper chest or outer arm or leg sites may be preferable although these too have their disadvantages. Catheters can be cumbersome but sexual intercourse is possible, particularly for women. Spigoting the catheter is usually less restricting and minimises pulling and therefore trauma. Spigoting may be uncomfortable for men, but a condom placed over the top of the occluded catheter can help to prevent friction and therefore bladder trauma. Leaving the catheter out for short periods, or intermittent suprapubic catheterisation, may be more acceptable.

Fungating wounds are possibly one of the most difficult issues for patients and partners to address as they can serve as a visual reminder of the disease process. Charcoal dressings and pleasant smelling essential oils can be useful. However it is important to bear in mind that a partner may not see the same things nurses and other healthcare workers see. A partner can see and love the whole person and all their history and experiences, and may therefore be less shocked than would be anticipated.

Becoming the carer

It would be remiss not to address the altered dynamics within a relationship caused by the dependency of one partner and the need for the other to become the main carer (see Chapter 14 for further discussion).

Transactional analysis (Berne, 1964) can be a helpful framework within which to view the changing dynamics of relationships where one partner is dying in that it suggests we all fulfil adult, child and parent roles. Long-term serious illness can force a partner towards a constant 'parent' role while the sick and cared-for partner is forced towards the 'child' role. In this situation the likelihood of the continuation or resumption of sexual activity becomes increasingly less likely – that one does not have sex with one's parent or child are generally accepted social dictates. Enabling partners to fulfil a more adult-to-adult relationship would perhaps facilitate sexual expression. Respite care is essential in this situation and, if it can be arranged, it can enable each partner to have time and space for him/herself. This can help them to detach from the parent or child role and prepare for a more adult sexual role. Individuals and couples may not understand these dynamics but a clearer understanding may be the route to a more fulfilling relationship.

Talking sex to angels

If openness is the key to successfully caring for people who are dying then we must consider the blocks that can exist to developing this kind of relationship with patients and their partners. The impact of the context of palliative care, in particular its inherent religious influences, has been explored. An added dimension is the perception that patients and partners may have of nurses, particularly those who work in palliative care. The perception of nurses as 'angels' has a long history (see Chapter 4) and, in addition, those who care for people who are dying are sometimes perceived with an almost sanctified status. It is difficult enough to raise issues of sexuality or sexual need, but perhaps even more so within a religious context where individuals are perceived to be 'pure', 'sanctified' or even 'angelic'.

'Permission' is the key and this can be offered in a range of forms – specific information that clearly states 'if there is anything you need to know please ask', and an environment that acknowledges the right of patients to discuss sexuality should they choose to do so, and one that is conducive to private discussion if this is required.

Giving 'permission', along with advice on creating the right situation, is one of the most affirming things that healthcare professionals can do – remembering that partners can support their loved one in life-affirming ways can help to make dying more a part of living. The following quote says more than I ever could to confirm this:

'In hospital we sit together waiting for his death. Holding his hand does not help. We are alienated because I can no longer come to him with the love and nourishment of my body. We always used sex as a means of easing the tension of the day and giving us sustenance for tomorrow. Now all is lost. I feel that I have been denied my right to help him in a way no one else can – in a way that no drug or doctor or nurse can help. Now I cannot ease his frustrations or give him proof of my love. I feel that I have abandoned him, that we are no longer facing his death together. I have failed him by letting his last days be away from home where there is no opportunity for physical closeness.'

(Siemens & Brandzel, 1982, p.47)

Conclusion

This chapter began by exploring the difficulties that can prevent healthcare professionals from talking to dying patients and concludes with some of the difficulties that dying patients may face in talking to healthcare professionals about sexuality. It aims to provoke thought about a difficult aspect of palliative care practice and to offer some suggestions for ways forward but, more importantly, to encourage practitioners to reflect upon their own practice setting and its impact on meeting patients' sexuality needs.

While I may have appeared critical of palliative care staff and services, as a former palliative care nurse, I am criticising myself. Years ago as a student nurse I can remember many times when I gave no thought at all to this important area of care. I remember vividly a dying man whom I cared for over a number of weeks. He made obvious his sexual needs but the nursing team met this situation with disgust. At no point did we consider his or his partner's needs and he died unable to receive or demonstrate passion, intimacy or commitment. This chapter is dedicated to him.

References

Berne, E. (1964) *Games People Play*. Penguin Books, London.

Biswas, B. (1993) In: D. Clarke (ed.) *The Future of Palliative Care – Issues of Policy and Practice*. Buckingham Press, Abingdon.

Cave, D. (1993) Chapter 58 in: D. Dickenson & M. Johnson (eds) *Death, Dying and Bereavement*. Sage, London.

Davenport-Hines, R. (1990) *Sex, Death and Punishment*. William Collins & Sons, Glasgow.

Gorden, G. (1966) *Role Theory and Illness*. New Haven College and University Press.

Griffin, S. (1981) *Pornography and Silence*. Harper & Row, New York.

Hollister, L. (1975) The mystique of social drugs and sex. In: M. Sandler & G. Gessa (eds) *Sexual Behaviour – Pharmacology and Biochemistry*. Raven, New York.

Hyde, J. (1994) *Understanding Human Sexuality*. McGraw-Hill, USA.

James, N. & Field, D. (1992) The routinisation of hospice: charisma and bureaucratisation. *Social Science and Medicine*, **34**, 12, 1363–75.

Pickering, M., Littlewood, J. & Walter, T. (eds) (1997) In: D. Field, J. Hockey & N. Small (eds) *Death, Gender and Ethnicity*. Routledge, London.

Rees, D. (1997) Death and Bereavement: The psychological, religious and cultural interfaces. Wurr Publishers, London.

Saunders, C. (1986) Hospices and services and AIDS victims. *The Times*, 2 August.

Savage, J. (1987) *Nurse Gender and Sexuality*. Heinemann Medical Books, London.

Schafer, M. & Olson, D. (1981) Assessing Intimacy – the PAIR inventory. *Journal of Marital and Family Therapy*, 47–60.

Siemens, S. & Brandzel, R. (1982) *Sexuality – Nursing Assessment and Intervention*. JB Lippincott, Philadelphia.

Stedeford, A. (1994) *Facing Death, Patients, Families and Professionals* (second edition). Sobell Publications, Oxford.

Sternberg, R.J. (1986) Theory of love. *Psychological Review*, **93**, 119–35.

Wasow, M. (1977) Human sexuality and terminal illness. *Health and Social Work*, **2**, 2, 105–21.

Worden, W. (1991) *Grief Counselling – Grief Therapy*. Springer, New York.

Part 3
Sexuality in Health and Illness

11. *Sexuality and People with Mental Health Needs*

Martin Ward

'Civilisation behaves toward sexuality as a people or a stratum of its population does (sic) which has subjected another one to its exploitation' (Gates, 1991). Here Gates was discussing the relationship between the psychoanalytical nature of culture and the complex issues surrounding racism. He was comparing philosophical thinking using Fanon, Greenblatt and Memmi, with the more psychodynamic processes associated with Freud. In doing so he managed to conjure up a place for sexuality within the social context that had hitherto only belonged to the more extreme forms of social abuse, such as racism, ageism and genderism. In identifying sexuality as a parallel to these complex social issues, and by placing it alongside others such as spirituality, it is easy to see why Apt *et al.* (1994) considered sexual behaviour to be the most under-researched of all human activities.

The aim of this chapter is to explore the nature and expression of sexuality, as it relates to mental health, in a more philosophical way than that usually associated with the subject. To this end I will compare sexuality and its expression with another phenomenon frequently oversimplified, that of racism. The reality within healthcare contexts is that sexuality, like racism, is often dealt with on a superficial or practical level. Too often, the focus may be permitting female patients to wear perfume or encouraging men to shave regularly, thus ignoring the whole process of self-expression and the psychology of power, control and dignity. To fully appreciate why individuals need to express their own sexuality, and not one contrived for them by others, it is necessary to have an understanding of self-worth, as illustrated by personal sexuality and to consider how this fits into the sociocultural jigsaw.

So, for those readers expecting to find ways of helping patients express their sexuality this is probably not the chapter to read. However if, like me, you feel that it is far more important to understand complex aspects of human expression in order to be better placed to consider the professional nursing response to them, it is hoped you will find the following chapter useful.

Sexuality and mental health

It is not so much mental health that interests us as mental ill health. Presumably an individual who has good mental health is self-fulfilling, has high self-esteem and worth, suffers little from the effects of stress and fatigue and is also able to express themselves satisfactorily. This may or may not be a correct assumption, for their sexuality may in fact be so dominant that it causes others to function less well and may, therefore, be deviant so far as society is concerned. However, we should consider the impact of poor sexual health functioning or sexual expression within the context of mental ill health.

Where an individual is incapable of identifying their place within the social order, cannot influence their day to day life satisfactorily, gets little or no satisfaction from contact with others and generally fails to achieve the realisation of their own needs, it is safe to assume that psychologically they will have difficulty maintaining a rewarding existence. Whatever else may be going on it is likely that mental ill health will either accompany these phenomena, or be the result of them.

Within the realms of mental illness the prevalence of sexuality as a major symptomatic constituent is not uncommon. Self-harm (Jones, 1996), violence (Koniac & Lesser, 1996), drug misuse (Alstron *et al.*, 1995), alcohol misuse (O'Hare, 1995), eating disorders (Rowston & Lacey, 1992) and schizophrenia (Lilleleht & Leiblum, 1993) are all examples of conditions or behavioural problems that have recognised elements of sexual expression within them.

For people who are mentally ill it is not just the conditions associated with mental ill health that can be associated with sexual expression. The structure of institutions and services may also have an impact upon the ability of an individual to express their sexuality. A dominating, suffocating environment would test even the most capable of individuals' ability to 'be' themselves. Given the fact that mental illness frequently reduces self-confidence and personal identity it is obvious that it would take an exceptional type of carer to be able both to identify the precise nature of a patient's sexuality deficit *and* to help them overcome it. In so much as nursing staff are often the first people who come into contact with patients accessing mental health services for problems associated with sexual expression, it is perhaps more important for nurses to be aware of the role they need to play in attempting to address such difficulties.

When taken to extremes you begin to realise that a nurse who is not comfortable in allowing others to express themselves fully is unlikely to enable a patient the potential return to mental health where their main problem also stems from problematic sexual expression. Those who appear mentally well themselves and who are therefore experiencing their own sexuality successfully, may not necessarily be therapeutic for those who are not so successful (Sharkey, 1997). As Purdie (1996) observes, the vulnerability of this healthcare group ought to be of particular concern for nurses, but if the nurse is either not alert to, or incapable of recognising, the features of sexual expression, it is difficult to see how this problem can be addressed.

The significance of being able to see the ways in which sexuality and its expression is used, both by the individual and by the society in which they perform, is a vital component of both self-awareness and the awareness of the needs of others. To appreciate fully how sexuality is used it is necessary to explore such concepts as power, control and self-actualisation.

Power and sexuality

To have power one must have individual forces, in this case human beings, where one can influence the other in some way. Hokansan Hawks (1991) maintains that there are two expressions of power, the 'power to' and the 'power over'. The first of these describes the ability of the individual to achieve goals but it is the second expression of power, the 'power over', which is of interest to us here.

In Finland, Raatikainen (1994) noted that 'powerful' nurses tended to be more knowledgeable, confident and were able to implement policies more often than powerless nurses. 'Power to' is at play here, but it might also be argued that if these powerful nurses did not act in such a way as to enable powerless nurses to achieve the same level of expression, then there may also be subtle evidence of 'power over'. Similarly, if nurses do not work in such a way as to enable patients to achieve self-determination then this could be seen as 'power over'. In other words, the 'power to' exerts pressure on the individual to have 'power over'. According to

171

Merton (1965) power is the predictable capacity for imposing one's self-will on social actions and, in this case, on the will of others. Powerlessness, conversely, is the unwillingness of an individual to accept such responsibility.

Traditional relationships within nursing are based upon the ability of the 'powerful' nurse to exert force upon the 'powerless' patient to comply with health giving practices and procedures. More recently, nursing has attempted to enter a more collaborative partnership with patients; the apparent purpose is an attempt to empower patients to take responsibility for certain aspects of their own care planning and delivery. However, there is evidence to suggest that when nurses appear to enable patients to make limited decisions for themselves, these decisions are actually based upon a set of options created by the nurse as a representative of the care team. This scenario simply reinforces nurses' control over the nurse–patient relationship and clinical arena (Porter, 1994). The nurse retains the 'power over', the patient assumes some responsibility for the 'power to', but only with the help of the nurse (Armstrong, 1983).

Sexuality, power and mental health nursing

The ability of one individual to exert power over another stems from their general knowledge and observations of the other. What those observations reveal will determine the communication that takes place between patient and nurse. It is therefore the nurse who determines the agenda, not the patient, even though the patient is the source of the information. In certain clinical settings, though perhaps less so in mental health, the nurse is also dealing with the power differentials between the knowledge of nurses, and the knowledge of doctors. If the doctor decides that information about a patient's mental state, risk factors and personal competence are an indication of their health status, then the nurse is bound to gather information about those elements. Therefore, what is meaningful within the patient–nurse relationship is predetermined by other forces outside the relationship itself. Consequently, the first paradox of the patient–nurse relationship is that its characteristics can be prescribed outside the relationship itself. Feelings and emotions are deemed relevant, but mainly when used to inform future decisions about treatments, medications and core programmes. One could argue that the acknowledgement of sexuality within this relationship may enable it to become more diverse, unique and thus more human.

Without the inclusion of sexuality as a force within the relationship the result is that lower care priorities, those which do not inform diagnostic or treatment strategies, often attract less 'real' communication time than those which conform with the healthcare team agenda. If nurses are unaware of the effects of sexuality and sexual expression upon a patient's perceived problems or behaviour, it is unlikely that such information will be moved from a lower to a higher priority status. If the knowledge to be known by the care team is centred upon behaviour alone, its antecedents remain unknown, and are thus more able to influence future behaviour unchecked.

No one would deny the underlying altruistic desires of nurses to improve the situation of their patients, but setting the priorities about how that is achieved is the essential power base of nurses, often under the influence of other powerful care team members (Dobes, 1990). Sexuality is a human quality and something that is also socially constructed. If the social context is more concerned with enabling mental health patients to conform to society's norms and values it is less likely to entertain elements which are fundamentally individual, and in this sense, deviant. Sexuality may fall into this category of meaning. Given that sexuality is the product of negotiation between one or more individuals and that its expression can be idiosyncratic in nature, it stands to reason that nurses dealing with other sets of priorities are unlikely to allow sexuality to enter into the observation equation. In this way sexuality remains outside the patient–nurse relationship or, if it does enter it, is only there because of its behavioural consequences and not its emotional importance to the patient.

The power of the patient–nurse relationship rests in trying to aggregate information so that it fits into what is already known about treatments and their effects. The power of the nurse rests within that knowledge. The power of human sexuality is therefore lost within the relationship simply because it is too personal. Therein lies the second paradox of the patient–nurse relationship. For mental health nursing to be successful it has to deny the very components of personal wellbeing which make up who the patient is, yet patients are expected to recover from their mental illness despite this failure to recognise who they are.

One other element needs to be considered here, that of the sexuality of the nurse. Nurses do not work in a social vacuum – their sexuality is socially constructed by their relationships with family, friends, other healthcare workers, and not solely their patients. It is that social construct which they bring to the patient–nurse relationship. Patients' expectations of the nurse within that relationship may be totally out of synchrony with what they actually receive. We are aware that often patients have a predetermined view of nurses and nursing. If patients do not get what they expect there may be a tendency for them to be disappointed and to take it personally. The rejection that may result could have serious consequences for both patient progress and nursing competence.

Ultimately, one has to make a link between the expression of a collaborative construction of one's sexuality and the 'power over' capabilities of another in permitting you to express your sexuality fully. If the nurse, through their traditional role within the care process, does not allow the patient to express that sexuality, that sense of 'self', the outcome can be a destructive or violent response. In effect, the nurse is saying that only the acceptable aspects of a patient's 'self' are important and this in turn devalues who the patient is. This may not happen at a conscious level, the patient does not say to him/herself 'I am very angry because you do not want to know who I really am or what I actually think', but the seeds of this frustration are sown. There is a feeling of denial and it is that feeling, that emotional response to the nurse, which is of such importance. No one can tell another how to feel, despite us often trying. We can perhaps suggest other ways of thinking or behaving, but not feeling because it is too fundamental and personal. An individual's sexuality is the storehouse of such feelings and when they are denied, undervalued, repressed or simply ignored, they are just as likely to produce as dramatic a consequence as any cognitive or behavioural antecedent.

The process is a progressive one; denial of sexual expression or denial of one's role and personal identity does not bring about an instant response. It will stay with an individual while they think about it, trying to understand why the nurse's response to them was not as they would have expected, why they don't appear to have been taken seriously, why their ideas are being ignored or discounted. Gradually they will begin to respond to the conclusions they reach and as this may take some time, the reaction that results may be totally out of context to the original cause. Thus, a patient may become angry and aggressive at a time when it seems totally inappropriate to do so, or their response to a single request from a nurse is hugely exaggerated. Such responses can represent a massive insult to the nurse's power base and subsequently may provoke heavy handed clinical responses. Perhaps the worst possible outcome is that the patient is trusted less and the relationship they had previously with the nurse becomes even less supportive. In reality, neither patient nor nurse benefits from denial of a patient's sexuality, but it is likely to be the patient who suffers most as a consequence of it.

Sexuality and the manifestation of oppression

To try to understand more of the relationship between sexuality, sexual expression, power and self-worth it is useful to explore a similar phenomenon, that of racism. Franz Fanon considered racism from a philosophical perspective; more specifically his work illustrated the possible stages that can be identified in the rejection of national identity. His work may have value for understanding the consequences of rejecting human sexuality within a mental health setting.

Sexuality, racism and the impact on mental health

Fanon, a psychiatrist and later a spokesperson for terrorist revolutionaries, believed that there were various stages that an oppressed people would go through before indulging in direct rebellion. Significantly, the sequence of behaviour he describes coincides directly with traditional theories of coercion. The parallels between Fanon's social psychology of racism and that of oppressed sexuality are:

- people who feel oppressed, either overtly or covertly, will initially tolerate such behaviour by others
- individuals move to a position whereby they try to resolve the situation by overemphasising their tolerance of others
- individuals begin to reject the oppression, or lack of recognition, through either non-compliance or an overexaggeration of their own responses to their feelings – in this case their own sexuality
- people finally resort to violence or violent outbursts.

The social psychology of Fanon, particularly as described by Adams (1970) and more recently by Hopton (1995) clearly locates the origins of mental distress in social injustice and oppression. While Fanon was seen by many political and professional observers simply as a violent radical (Robinson, 1993), within his works is the recognition that people will eventually always rebel against perceived injustice, no matter how subtle that injustice may be.

Fanon (1965) shows us that sexuality too may well be locked into the oppression and injustice paradigm. The marked similarities between failure to recognise someone's racial identity and someone's sexual identity are clear to see. Hopton (1995) also explores the problem associated with power relations between patient and

175

nurse, endorsing Fanon's belief that the oppressor does not always seem to be the main cause of the oppression. Nurses do not necessarily ignore the sexuality of their patients, they may simply devalue it, or place a lower order of priority upon it. The 'oppressor' in this case is actually quite benign but may receive the full force of the patient's anger as they reach the end of their tolerance for such rejection.

Mental health practice: the lesson to be learned

The most significant comparison between sexuality and racism is that no one seems prepared to discuss either in any depth at a clinical level. A review of the mental health literature reveals that the evidence base related to sexuality is relatively sparse, with Payne and Hardy (1993), Bhui and Puffett (1994) and Park Dorsay and Forchuk (1994) being notable exceptions. The application of Fanon's approach to oppression to the concept of sexuality in mental health care suggests that mental health nurses need more than assessment and diagnostic tools to be able to deal effectively with their patients' unique expression of sexuality. Nurses must be able both to appreciate the fundamental need for recognition of the complexities of sexual identity that are related to self-expression and to be able to appreciate their own beliefs, values and prejudices in relation to the subject. The analysis of Fanon's work also gives us something else: it enables us to say that sexuality and its expression is rooted within the social context and may be heavily influenced by the degree of 'power over' that an individual possesses to be themselves. Fanon also gives us some insight into what may be the negative outcomes if an individual's sexuality is not given an appropriate outlet.

Finally, if people do not feel that they are understood and if their needs are not being met, eventually they will do something about it no matter how passive or compliant they appear to be. Patients experiencing severely handicapping mental health problems may not have the appropriate skills to be able to access their 'power over' strength and will therefore be more likely to react strongly to their need recognition. Unlike those experiencing racism, patients may not actually know what it is that is making them angry, which in turn may make the situation worse. All individuals may feel is a sense of injustice, powerlessness or a feeling of being devalued. Whatever the cause, the consequence will be the same – destructive communication between patient and nurse, a resultant increase in the 'power over' response from the nurse, with a possible escalation of inappropriate behaviour from the patient. Nobody wins, everybody loses, but it is the patient who loses most.

Conclusion

Sexuality is a personal signature that is accompanied by feelings of worth and self-esteem. The ability to express sexuality will be dictated by the power an individual has within a given setting: the more powerful they are, the more they will be able to express themselves. In mental health services the ability to express sexuality may often depend upon the facilitative capabilities of the nurse, and their willingness and skill to recognise the patients' need to do so. Once expressed, a patient's sexuality has to be taken seriously and treated as a priority issue. Failure to do so may well result in anger and violence.

Through comparison of the issues of racism and sexuality it is possible to detect a behavioural continuum, with self-expression and contentment at one end and dissatisfaction and distress at the other. We can clarify our understanding of sexuality by recognising that oppression, in this case of a person's sexual identity, will almost certainly generate a feeling of injustice which in turn will eventually surface in hostile behaviour towards the identified oppressor.

It is necessary for mental health nurses to develop an understanding of their own sexual tolerances, their own feelings and beliefs about the way they express them and their expectation of others in allowing them the opportunity to do so. In turn they have to provide the time and space for their patients to do exactly the same thing. Lingis (1994) described how a person told how beautiful they were did not respond by simply accepting elements of themselves they already knew about, they would re-create or re-recognise themselves in the knowledge that someone else saw this within them. Such a response would, more often than not, produce a smile. Whilst I am not suggesting that mental health nurses should simply go around telling their patients they all look beautiful, I do think that being positive towards an individual's sexuality might be the first step towards understanding the nature of that sexuality and sharing the power to express it.

References

Adams, P.L. (1970) The social psychiatry of Franz Fanon. *American Journal of Psychiatry*, **127**, 6, 809–14.

Alstron, R.J., Harley, D. & Lenhoff, K. (1995) Hirschi's social control theory:

a sociological perspective on drug abuse among persons with disabilities. *Journal of Rehabilitation*, **61**, 4, 31–5.

Apt, C., Hurlbert, D.F. & Clark, K.J. (1994) Neglected subjects in sex research and survey of sexologists. *Journal of Sex and Marital Therapy*, **20**, 3, 237–43.

Armstrong, D. (1983) The fabrication of nurse–patient relationships. *Social Science and Medicine*, **17**, 8, 457–60.

Bhui, K. & Puffett, A. (1994) Sexual problems in the psychiatric and mentally handicapped populations. *British Journal of Hospital Medicine*, **51**, 9, 459–64.

Dobes, C.L. (1990) Big fish in a big pool: empowerment, assertiveness and risk taking among nurses. *Today's OR Nurse*, **12**, 8, 12–16.

Fanon, F. (1965) *The Wretched of the Earth* (Trans. C. Farrington). Grove Press, New York.

Gates, H.L. (1991) Critical Fanonism. *Critical Enquiry*, Spring, 457–70.

Hokansan Hawks, J. (1991) Power: a concept analysis. *Journal of Advanced Nursing*, **16**, 754–62.

Hopton, J. (1995) The application of the ideas of Franz Fanon to the practice of mental health nursing. *Journal of Advanced Nursing*, **21**, 723–8.

Jones, A. (1996) An equal struggle: psychodynamic assessment following repeated episodes of deliberate self-harm. *Nursing*, **3**, 3, 173–80.

Koniak, G.D. & Lesser, J. (1996) The impact of childhood maltreatment on young mothers' behaviour towards themselves and others. *Nursing*, **11**, 5, 300–308.

Lilleleht, E. & Leiblum, S.R. (1993) Schizophrenia and sexuality: a critical review of the literature. *Annual Review of Sex Research*, **4**, 247–76.

Lingis, A. (1994) *Faces, Idols and Fetishes*, p.48. Indiana University Press, Bloomington and Indiana.

Merton, R.K. (1965) *Social Theory and Social Structure*. The Free Press, New York.

O'Hare, T. (1995) Mental health problems and alcohol abuse: Co-occurrence and gender differences. *Health and Social Work*, **20**, 3, 207–14.

Park Dorsay, J. & Forchuk, C. (1994) Assessment of the sexuality needs of individuals with psychiatric disability. *Journal of Psychiatric and Mental Health Nursing*, **1**, 93–7.

Payne, A. & Hardy, S. (1993) Sexual activity among psychiatric inpatients: international perspectives – England. *Journal of Forensic Psychiatry*, **4**, 1.

Porter, S. (1994) New nursing: the road to freedom? *Journal of Advanced Nursing*, **20**, 269–74.

Purdie, H. (1996) Management of sexuality in mental health settings. *Nursing Standard*, **11**, 12, 7–50.

Raatikainen, R. (1994) Power or the lack of it in nursing care. *Journal of Advanced Nursing*, **19**, 424–32.

Robinson, C. (1993) The appropriation of Franz Fanon. *Race and Class*, **35**, 1, 79–91.

Rowston, W.M. & Lacey, J.H. (1992) Stealing in bulimia nervosa. *International Journal of Social Psychiatry*, **38**, 4, 309–13.

Sharkey, V.B. (1997) Sexuality, sexual abuse. Omissions in admissions? *Journal of Advanced Nursing*, **25**, 5, 1025–32.

12. Sexuality and People Affected by Sexually Transmitted Infections

Elizabeth Grigg

Our knowledge of the range of sexually transmitted infections (STIs) has widened greatly since the early 1980s. The incidence of syphilis and gonorrhoea continues to rise and in some countries gonorrhoea is encountered in epidemic proportions, even though it is treatable if recognised. Other STIs caused by chlamydia trachomatis, the human papilloma virus (HVP), genital herpes, the human immuno-deficiency virus (HIV) and non-specific urethritis (NSU) have also become major problems in the UK and in the rest of the world.

Infections caused by sexual contact evoke feelings of deep embarrassment and shame in many people and because they mostly involve the genital area they are also associated with privacy and intimacy. Health professionals involved in sexual health care have to be expert practitioners and be able to deal with some of the most sensitive issues affecting human beings. In 1932 Lucy Seymer wrote of tuberculosis nursing and venereal disease nursing as constituting 'special parts of public health work'. These infectious diseases were defined as posing a 'deadly danger to the community'. She stated that: 'Tuberculosis is overwhelmingly the greatest cause of death and sickness – as to the other diseases, special training for the prompt recognition of the evil is eminently desirable' (Seymer, 1932, p.217).

However, despite increased public health education about STIs and legal structures to prevent their spread, these infections are increasing both in type and in incidence. Moreover they will continue to be out of control as long as the secrecy, prompted by the bigotry that surrounds them, remains (Western, 1999). Throughout history they have been, and continue to be, associated with immorality, 'unclean living', 'evil acts' and prostitution (Morton, 1976). Women have been, and remain, frequently portrayed as the perpetrators.

A brief history of STIs: BC–1900 AD

Gonorrhoea

The earliest references to a disease that was possibly gonorrhoea are cited in the Bible. In Leviticus XV, God tells Moses and Aaron that a man suffering a urethral discharge should be regarded as unclean (Morton, 1976). Moses apparently recognised that the disease was transmitted by sexual contact and promoted a sexual health regimen for the Israelites. This included the need for washing after sexual intercourse, a seven day quarantine for men who might have 'lain' with women from Midian and the killing of Midianite women prisoners who might have 'lain' with men and were thus a source of infection.

Despite such drastic measures, infections continued and King David himself lamented that his loins 'were filled with a loathsome disease' (Morton, 1976, p.117). Similarly in Hindu and Chinese mythology, diseases caused by sexual contact are cited. In 400 AD a specific mention is made in Hindu writings of a disease which produced 'unhealthy humours in the penis' and was caused by contact with a woman's vulva.

In Britain the first citation of gonorrhoea was in a London Act of 1161, which forebade brothel keepers employing 'women suffering from the perilous suffering of burning' (Morton, 1976, p.117).

The Frenchman John of Arderne first coupled the word 'clap' with the burning disease in 1378. Clap was part of Paris then frequented by female prostitutes. In 1430 the term 'the hidden disease' was used in London and authorities forbade men who suffered from this affliction admittance to brothels.

The word 'venereal' derives from the Latin *venerius*, to do with Venus the goddess of love, and still remains the legal term for both gonorrhoea and syphilis in some countries. Although displaying different symptoms, syphilis was not recognised as a different disease until the end of the eighteenth century. Early in the eighteenth century, at a time when 'it is hardly one chance in ten that a Town Spark of that age has not been clapt' (Morton, 1976, p.118), a surgeon by the name of John Hunter suggested that the different symptoms depended on where the infection entered the body. To prove this he inoculated himself with the pus of an infected man.

Unfortunately, the man was suffering from both gonorrhoea and syphilis. John Hunter's experiment proved worthless and he eventually died of the late stages of syphilis.

In 1873 Benjamin Bell finally proved the existence of two distinct diseases by conducting experiments on his medical students. In 1879, shortly after the introduction of the microscope, the *neisseria gonorrhoease* (meaning seed) *or gonococcus bacterium* was isolated as the cause of gonorrhoea. Many thousands of people suffered from its consequences. It commonly caused blindness in babies and sterility and debilitating arthritic conditions in adults, and still does if untreated.

In 1936 sulphonamides brought about the first effective cure but within ten years sulphonamide-resistant strains of the disease developed. Although at present gonorrhoea is treated effectively with antibiotics its incidence continues to rise.

Syphilis

Knowledge about syphilis appears to date back to the fifteenth century when an epidemic swept through Europe. It is not clear from where it originated, although one theory is that it was carried from the Americas by Christopher Columbus and his crew when they returned from their voyage of discovery (Hastings, 1974). Another theory is that it is a form of the disease yaws, which is common in the tropics. Its bacteria live on the hot sweaty skin of its host. It was theorised that slaves imported from Africa could have brought it to Europe and the yaws organisms had to adapt to survive and moved to the warm genital, anal and oral areas of their host and were thus transmitted by sexual contact.

The third theory is that the two diseases appeared simultaneously but yaws died out in Europe because of increasing knowledge about hygiene in the fifteenth century. According to Morton (1976) the first major appearance of syphilis was amongst the Spanish and French soldiers of both sides during the siege of Naples in 1495. A Portuguese physician had previously treated some of Columbus's men in Barcelona with a disease, which he called 'Indian Measles'. He was later to state that this was the same disease.

Syphilis played havoc amongst the French soldiers, causing Charles VIII of France to abandon his campaign and disperse his army. The men carried the disease to the rest of Europe. It reached Paris in 1496, London in 1497 and was recognised in Scotland as sexually transmitted in the same year. In 1498 it reached India and in 1505 it had reached China. Each country blamed another: it was called 'the French pox' by the Germans and the English, 'the Italian disease' by the French and the 'Portuguese sickness' by the Japanese. The name syphilis arises from a poem written by an Italian physician, Girolama Fracastoro in 1530. The hero Syphilis offended the god Apollo and was therefore struck down by a terrible disease similar to the one raging through Europe at the time.

During the first hundred years of the disease's existence many thousands of people died. It was extremely virulent with rashes, mouth, nose and throat ulcers, bone pain and high fever. By the seventeenth century it appeared that people had become more resistant, the disease was less obvious and early death was unlikely (Morton, 1976).

Treatment varied from prayer and isolation to the application of mercury, which was rubbed into the skin, inhaled or taken by mouth. Mercury had long been used for skin conditions but was as dangerous as the disease itself. William Wallace introduced potassium iodide, which is still occasionally used today. In 1905 the physicians Fritz Shaudinn and Eric Hoffmann discovered the organism that causes syphilis: *treponema pallidum* and in 1906 August von Wasserman developed a blood test that made diagnosis more certain. Treatment then consisted of arsenic preparations, which were highly effective and only superseded by the discovery of penicillin by Sir Alexander Fleming.

Antibiotics brought the incidence of both syphilis and gonorrhoea under control, despite its prevalence during more recent wars. However, both diseases and other STIs can no longer be linked to outbreaks of war, nor can they always be linked to poverty (Farmer, 1999).

The secret diseases of prosperity

Many notable people throughout history have been affected by STIs. Morton (1976) cites examples such as Louis XIV of France, Edward VII of Britain and James Boswell, the biographer of Samuel Johnson, with gonorrhoea; Henry VIII suffered from syphilis. Artists, writers and musicians, such as Guy de Maupassant, Dostoevsky, Charles Baudelaire and Gauguin became insane as a result of syphilis. Molière and Schumann died from it and Beethoven's deafness was possibly caused by congenital syphilis. Van Gogh, Ivan the Terrible, Lenin, Napoleon and eminent churchmen, such as Cardinals Richelieu and Wolsey, who enjoyed enormous worldly power, all suffered from STIs.

In 1770, Catherine the Great of Russia established the first hospital devoted to the treatment of venereal diseases. Other countries followed suit, driven by the reluctance among traditional hospitals to treat socially unacceptable diseases. In Britain they were known as lock hospitals.

Even today, care for people with diseases that have sexual connotations often remains distinct from the mainstream of healthcare provision. Clinics to deal exclusively with STIs have emerged, not because of the specialism *per se*, but because of the complex social and emotional need for these diseases to be kept 'hidden' from mainstream medicine.

With the advent of the HIV which, in Western society, involved gay men, drug users and people perceived to be on the moral fringes of society, hospitals were given specific extra funding to provide separate clinical areas for people with Acquired Immuno-deficiency Syndrome (AIDS).

The Genito-Urinary Medicine Clinic

The first Special Clinics to deal with STIs were set up in 1916. Treatment was free at the point of delivery and remains so. However, the name Special Clinic was embarrassingly associated with sex and in some hospitals these clinics were given a ward number or name to ensure confidentiality and alleviate the humiliation people may have felt by associating themselves with such clinics. Despite such attempts, these clinics were known locally as the 'the VD clinic', 'the clap clinic' or 'the pox clinic'.

In the 1980s the name Genito-Urinary Medicine Clinic (GUM) followed. This is a name that arguably does not reflect the conditions it deals with and one that causes confusion to both patients and healthcare workers. There are incidences of dental clinics being near to GUM clinics. In the UK the number of people visiting GUM clinics has risen over fourfold since the early 1980s with over 800,000 new cases a year (Adler, 1995), the greatest increase being in women patients.

These clinics still remain embarrassing for patients to visit and can be difficult for nurses to work in (Grigg, 1997). Bromelow (1990) was told by her tutor that working with STIs was not 'proper nursing'. Around the world GUM clinics are typically hidden from public view and are often situated in the basement of hospitals, near the boilers or the mortuary, or at the back of local authority health departments. Externally they are usually most unwelcoming for both patients and staff, while internally they are frequently cramped and at the bottom of the health authority refurbishment budget.

This sort of location serves to reinforce the clandestine nature of infections caused by intimate contact. However, some people are extremely grateful that the clinics are concealed from public sight and that they can visit them with privacy. It helps to ensure the confidentiality that GUM clinics guarantee. Confidentiality of treatment was established, and is maintained, by the Venereal Disease Act of 1974. In some areas GUM clinics are now called Sexual Health Clinics and have combined with Sexual Health and Contraception Clinics (formerly Family Planning Clinics (FPA)).

In urban areas people have access to Well Women clinics or Well Men clinics. However, many people do not have access to these services and have to visit their general practitioner (GP) for treatment. For some people this may be difficult, particularly in small communities, where the GP may be a family friend. The guilt, shame and blame that surround infections with sexual connotations makes seeking treatment difficult anyway. It takes an enormous amount of courage to access help in a locality where anonymity is not guaranteed – arguably especially for the young, but also for anyone who risks being labelled by their community as deviant through 'catching' an STI.

STIs are as complex as sexuality itself, the diseases are changing as well as increasing in incidence. The occurrence of infections has appeared to reflect changing attitudes towards sex throughout history. However, increasing infection and treatment brings about resistance to diseases, the organisms change and mutate and continually provide a challenge both to medicine and to care.

The changing emphasis of the diseases: 1900–the present day

Although gonorrhoea is still one of the most common STIs and its incidence is increasing amongst the young, non-specific genital infection and the genital wart virus will possibly cause more severe, long-term, lasting effects in this section of the population. Many young people have not heard of chlamydia or know about the effects of genital warts. It seems that they are far more concerned about the consequences of an unplanned pregnancy, which arguably is not as life threatening as many STIs.

Non-specific urethritis (NSU) caused by chlamydia and genital warts, in turn caused by the papilloma virus, is increasing at an alarming rate. Increases in medical knowledge, the availability of sophisticated technology and enhanced communication channels have done nothing substantial to control the spread of STIs and to change human behaviour in the area of sexuality and risk.

Genital warts

It has been stated that treating genital warts in GUM clinics is 'the "bread and butter" of the clinic'. However over 80% of cases are treated by GPs, dermatologists and gynaecologists. In the UK there are about 90,000 new cases a year (Adler, 1995). Genito-anal warts have been known about for centuries, the ancient Greeks gave them the name *condylomata* meaning knuckle and the name *ficus* meaning fig was also commonly used.

In 1954 they were recognised as being sexually transmitted and frequently observed in the wives of American soldiers who had served in the Korean War. In 1969 the human papilloma virus (HPV) was found in genital warts but it was not until 1980 that molecular biology techniques determined that there were many different types.

Genital warts are caused by a small DNA virus belonging to the papavirus group and they differ from skin warts both histologically and antigenically. They are almost entirely transmitted by sexual contact and hand to genital infection is rare. The infectivity of sexually acquired warts is 60%, the incubation period varies from two weeks to eight months. However 50% of infected people remain asymptomatic and women are more likely to be unaware of warts because it is harder for them to examine their genitals.

HPV may also remain dormant in the epithelium without inducing macroscopic or microscopic changes. Genital warts can occur wherever sexual contact occurs, but can also occur in areas where there has not been direct sexual contact. They may be solitary but are usually multiple by the time people present for treatment. Warts flourish in warm, moist conditions particularly if a discharge or other infections are present. Even when the lesions are not visible they actively produce and shed virus particles that are readily transmissible. Lesions can occur in the urethra where they are an unseen reservoir of disease and papilloma viral DNA has been found in the semen of men afflicted with chronic wart disease (Roberts, 1987).

The advent of rapid changes throughout the western world and an increased spatial mobility of susceptible populations have been well documented. It was suggested several years ago that the upsurge of STIs would predict a commensurate upswing in the number of women who were at risk of developing cancer of the lower genital tract. There are over 50 different types of HVP, most types appearing to cause only benign disease. Of the viruses involved in genital disease, types 6 and 11 cause typical genital warts and seem to be relatively harmless, but types 16 and 18 consistently show up in cellular dysplasia and cervical cancer. Results show that 80 to 90% of cancer and precursor lesions in the lower genital tract of young women contain the hallmark of HPV. In 1986 Professor Martin Tattersall described cervical cancer as the female equivalent of AIDS. Certainly people who are immuno-compromised are susceptible to HPV infection.

There are studies of men who have remarried after their first wife has died of cervical cancer that indicate their second wife has twelve times the normal risk of developing the same malignancy. There is also some evidence that the papilloma virus may be associated with cancer of the penis, the vulva and the vagina.

HPV has also been linked to a heritable skin disease and in 25% of people with this condition, ultimately to squamous carcinoma of the nongenital skin (Baird, 1986). Infants and children can be affected by laryngeal papillomas from maternal infection at delivery.

It was not until the late 1970s that macroscopically invisible flat warts on the cervix were linked to the high incidence of cervical preneoplasia found in a younger age group of women than previously. Vulval preneoplasia had been regarded traditionally as a postmenopausal disease.

The increase in incidence of genital warts is not necessarily a disease of promiscuity of women. Monogamous women are hostage to the sexual behaviour of their partners. In Columbia the incidence of cervical carcinoma reached epidemic proportions in the late 1980s, yet virginity is obligatory for Columbian brides. The cancer may have been linked to the almost mandatory promiscuity, chiefly with prostitutes, of young Columbian men (Roberts, 1987).

Globally, cervical cancer remains one of the leading causes of morbidity and death among women. Cervical cancer classically develops slowly, only materialising 10 to 20 years after the initial insult, but virulent precancerous growths are emerging that can turn malignant in a matter of months. In the late 1960s only 1% of all cases involved women under 35 years of age, yet in the 1990s they accounted for over 30%. In Australia, in 1986, it was estimated that 30% of women who reach 35 will have HPV or abnormal cervical cells associated with the virus and the incidence is rising.

An increase in the incidence of carcinoma of the cervix, coupled with the virulent disease that is associated with rapidly developing lesions in multiple sites could be linked to the variations of viral virulence. Variations of viral virulence are well known in microbiology, they are unusually assigned to mutations in the viral genetic apparatus. It has been postulated that HPV changes, strengthens and becomes more carcinogenic as it moves from host to host through sexual contact (Baird, 1986).

Treatment can be arduous and time consuming, with initial treatment normally comprising a locally applied caustic agent two or three times per week. Attending for treatment can be socially difficult but it is undesirable for patients to treat themselves as the agents can burn if applied incorrectly and it is very tempting for people to overdose to get rid of the 'growths' on their body that they perceive as 'disgusting'.

Larger and more resistant lesions may require cauterisation or surgical excision. Warts can regress spontaneously and some people have recurrent episodes of infection without associated sexual contact; treatment efficacy is thus difficult to evaluate.

All women attending for treatment should be encouraged to have cytology performed at least every year and all sexually active women, irrespective of their sexual activity, should be encouraged to attend for cervical smears at least every second year. Screening for carcinoma of the cervix is arguably cheaper than treating it. Screening for other diseases should also be a priority in public health. Chlamydia trachomatis is the most common curable STI in the UK and early detection and treatment can prevent irreparable damage.

Chlamydia trachomatis

Peter Tatham stated that when he worked in a VD clinic during the early 1960s one saw a great deal of what was then called non-gonoccal urethritis (NGU), presenting as a painful discharge in the male and any female partner usually being without symptoms. It definitely followed sexual intercourse and it usually cleared up with a regimen of antibiotics, no sex and no alcohol. According to Tatham, the majority of people treated at clinics for STIs in the 1980s were diagnosed as having this same non-specific genital infection. Chlamydia trachomatis has been isolated as causing 50 to 70% of NGU in men. It is symptomless in 25% of cases but for 75% of men it causes dysuria and a mucoid discharge from the penis. Symptoms are usually less marked than with gonococcal urethritis but diagnosis should not be made purely on clinical grounds.

Chlamydia trachomatis can cause epididymo-orchitis in young sexually active young men and it has been linked to prostatitis. In one study chlamydia trachomatis was detected in 20 out of 45 men with non-bacterial prostatitis. Furthermore 48% of their female partners were found to have chlamydia trachomatis in early morning urine specimens (McMillan & Scott, 1991).

It has been mooted that chlamydia infection affects at least 5% of sexually active women and 80% of them will never know that they have it until they discover they cannot have children. Chlamydia trachomatis may be implicated in 50% of pelvic inflammatory disease (PID) including salpingitis, tubal obstruction, ectopic pregnancy and infertility.

The chlamydia bacterium has a 48-hour life cycle, which presents problems for both testing and therapy, and it takes only one invasion of chlamydia trachomatis to cause salpingitis. Women who have had three attacks have a 75% chance of being infertile. Studies show that 15% of women with chlamydial PID fail to respond to treatment and 20% will have at least one recurrence. The lifestyle and sexual activity of a woman is significant. It has been observed that PID is sexually transmitted in almost all cases in western society. Estimates from the United States of America and Europe from the late 1970s suggest that the annual incidence of PID in women of 15–24 years of age rose from 13 cases per 1000 to 20 cases per 1000 in the 1990s. In the USA, during the 1990s, the incidence of ectopic pregnancies had quadrupled (Weisburg, 1992). Chlamydial PID has less severe and obvious symptoms than gonoccal PID and therefore women are less likely to attend for treatment and more likely to develop infertility.

Chlamydia infection also appears to be the most prevalent paediatric STI. First, in neonates from their mothers during delivery, second, because of the early onset of sexual activity in the young and third because of child sexual abuse (Hill, 1990). Chlamydial infections in the very young have serious sequelae. Chlamydiae are bacteria that have many of the characteristics of a virus and there are uncertainties about them which are intriguing.

Sometimes chlamydiae can be cultured from the genital tract of people who have no disease and some female partners are found to be clear even if the male is infected. Males can suffer a recurrence and sometimes they will present with a non-specific urethritis, with no chlamydial infection, but chlamydia will be cultured from their partner's genitalia.

It is vital that couples are treated concurrently even if one partner is not showing positive. Failure to recognise the sexually transmitted aetiology of the disease can result in repeated infection of the patient and inadequate control of its spread in the community. Of all the social methods available for limiting the spread of STIs, the most direct and effective is the tracing and treating of all the sexual contacts of an infected person.

However, health professionals must understand that the issue of post STI contact tracing, treatment and safer sexual practices are extremely problematic. For example, some people may find it impossible to negotiate safer sexual practices with their partners after they have been diagnosed with an STI. There may be many reasons for this. They may not have previously even talked about sex in their relationship, making discussion about precautions embarrassing and probably impossible. Some people may have contracted the infection outside a permanent relationship and any disclosure could be a trigger for abuse, threat or relationship breakdown. Moreover, many people are reluctant and fear retribution should any contact be made with the person who infected them, whether this is a regular partner or a casual affair. Furthermore, experience from GUM clinics indicates that many people do not actually know who infected them.

Chlamydia trachomatis has been called 'the silent disease'; its lack of noticeable symptoms do not help in controlling its growing threat to people's health. Routine screening for all sexually active women must take place. GUM and FPA clinics are increasingly carrying this out, but many GP surgeries are not. Unless all healthcare providers offer routine screening, diseases caused by chlamydial infection and the papilloma virus will continue to spread.

Other infections

The epidemiology of STIs throughout history has varied but STIs have never been obliterated. All STIs, even though some are less damaging in the long term than others, should be investigated and treated seriously, as they may be a signpost for other more serious conditions. All STIs can present concurrently with other STIs.

Non-gonoccocal urethritis (NGU) is a urethral discharge (in males) not caused by gonorrhoea; NSU is the diagnosis for all those non-gonoccal infections of the urethra (in males) not caused by chlamydia trachomatis. Accurate microbiological tests are essential to eliminate gonorrhoea and chlamydia trachomatis, as antibiotic treatment differs. Unfortunately, 50% of men will be asymtomatic. Interestingly, 30% of their partners will have chlamydia trachomatis, while 10% of their partners will develop PID although negative to chlamydia trachomatis. NSU can be caused by candidiasis or could be activated by bacterial vaginosis in a partner.

Bacterial vaginosis or non-specific vaginitis is induced by an imbalance in the acid in the vagina and may be caused by spermatozoa or bacteria. Infections such as vaginal candidiasis (caused by fungi), which affects 75% of women, vaginal trichomoniasis (caused by protozoa) and which is implicated in other STIs, and infestations such as pediculosis pubis and scabies can all be transmitted sexually and are often seen in GUM clinics. They have been known about for some time and treatment is successful.

Most people have heard of herpes and 75% of people are infected with herpes simplex viruses with a continued increase in incidence. Type 2 causes genital or anal ulceration. Some people do not know that they are infected and may never present with an ulcer, but they can still be infectious, other people will develop extremely painful ulceration. Anti-viral treatment is usually effective in the primary stages but not so if the ulcers reoccur. Herpes can have a detrimental influence on some people's quality of life but is not life threatening in adults, while maternal to neonatal infection is 70% fatal. However, herpes sores may be a symptom of other diseases such as HIV or they could be confused with a syphilitic chancre.

Some of the hepatitis viruses can also be transmitted sexually. Hepatitis B and C are serious infections and hepatitis C is increasingly found amongst people who do not practise risk reduction and harm minimisation when using intravenous drugs. Hepatitis C has also been linked to HIV (Pratt, 1995).

There are many well documented issues that concern HIV and AIDS (Pratt, 1995). The new combination therapy treatment for HIV is having a profound impact upon the progression of the disease in the western world. How this will affect the future of the disease and those infected is not known but the global incidence continues to rise and to elicit panic, fear and prejudice from people in the same way as syphilis did in the sixteenth century.

The future

Despite our so-called 'permissive society', any illness that has sexual implications is still looked upon by many with intolerance. Nonetheless, all people are sexual beings and will express their sexuality in whatever ways they choose, and have done so throughout history. As Bancroft (1989, p.1) states 'The thread of sexuality is woven into the fabric of human existence'. Whilst few would argue with Bancroft's view, the total concept of sexuality is complex and remains ill understood. It is still not clear which sexual behaviours or expressions of sexuality are biologically determined and which are culturally driven. What is clear is that it is rare for people in any society not to have been influenced by sex during some part of their lives; for some it plays a crucial part. Sex brings people together in intimate contact but not always for reproduction.

Intimacy is not necessarily biologically driven, in fact in human beings and in some primates, sex has a socially cohesive role.

Given the complexity of sexuality it is not surprising that the subject is surrounded with difficulties, lack of understanding and knowledge, misunderstanding, prejudice and confusion. Human beings are vulnerable to sexual problems and are stigmatised by other humans if they do not conform to what is perceived as 'normal' or 'healthy' in society at that time. There is a powerful link between sexual 'normality' or attractiveness, sexual health and self-esteem (Bancroft, 1989).

The incidence and variety of STIs is on the increase and of great concern to western society are those diseases which are not well known, but are intensifying enough to have a huge impact on populations and their future health. Not only will this have cost implications within healthcare provision and services but also the consequences of these infections could have devastating effects on an individual's quality of life (Farmer, 1999).

Legal, moral, social and medical endeavours have not been successful in controlling STIs. Perhaps the only way to stem their flow is through research aimed at the development of vaccination and immunisation techniques. That process has been effective with diseases such as poliomyelitis, measles and diphtheria, which are also spread by social contact. When STIs are widely accepted simply as diseases, and not associated with prejudice, intolerance and diverse sexual acts, then society will have a much better chance to manage their control. Without general acceptance many people will continue to hide their conditions, even from their sexual partners, and STIs will continue to multiply. Surely what makes humanity unique and valuable lies both in our diversity and in our willingness to embrace all our consensual states of desire.

References

Adler, M. (1995) *ABC of Sexually Transmitted Diseases* (third edition). BMJ Publications, London.

Baird, P.J. (1986) Papilloma (wart) virus and cervical cancer. *Healthright*, **5**, 3, 8.

Bancroft, J. (1989) *Human Sexuality and its Problems* (second edition). Churchill Livingstone, Edinburgh.

Bromelow, I. (1990) Special Contracts. *Nursing Times*, **86**, 20, 48–9.

Farmer, P. (1999) *Infections and Inequalities*. University of California Press, Berkeley.

Grigg, E.M. (1997) A situational analysis of an HIV/AIDS clinical area. *Journal of Clinical Nursing*, **6**, 35–41.

Hastings, P. (1974) *Medicine: an International History*. Ernest Benn, London.

Hill, T. (1990) Chlamydia: most prevalent sexual infection in adolescents. *Australian Doctor*, September.

McMillan, A. & Scott, G.R. (1991) *Sexually Transmitted Diseases*. Churchill Livingstone, London.

Morton, R.S. (1976) Venereal diseases. In: *Encyclopaedia of Love and Sex*, pp.118–21. Marshall Cavendish, New York.

Pratt, R. (1995) *AIDS: A Strategy for Nursing Care*. Edward Arnold, London.

Roberts, L. (1987) Sex and cancer. *Issues in Science and Technology*, May.

Seymer, L.R. (1932) *A General History of Nursing*. Faber & Faber, London.

Weisburg, E. (1992) Pelvic inflammatory disease: an overview. *Healthright*, **5**, 4, 18–24.

Western, A. (1999) *Sexually Transmitted Infections*. Nursing Times Books, London.

Sexuality and People with Acute Illness

Danny Kelly

Depending on the nature of the illness involved, the focus of nursing in acute care may be seen to span a broad continuum from observing and caring for totally dependent patients in highly technical environments, e.g. intensive care, to preparing someone admitted for minor day case surgery to return home. When this diversity of role is considered it becomes clear that acute illness, as a term, has an enormous range of meanings. The reader is therefore invited to examine the key issues raised by this chapter and to consider their relevance to both individual practice and to acute care settings.

The changing awareness of sexuality in acute illness

A new awareness has developed of issues related to holistic care, including human sexuality, which are relevant for consideration by nursing. If sexuality is ignored, the health care offered to patients may be far from holistic. Instead, care is at risk of being fragmented and confined to those accepted routines and rituals that are considered 'safe' and do not threaten to disrupt the sensitive boundaries between the parties involved (Lawler, 1991). During periods of acute ill health, therefore, the importance of sexuality requires re-examination in order to appreciate its relevance.

Within western models of health care, acute illness is firmly located within a dominant biomedical paradigm which views the body as a series of interdependent physiological systems which have the capacity to malfunction (Armstrong, 1987; Turner, 1987; Elston, 1991; Fox, 1995). Nursing theory, operating from within the influences of this biomedical culture, claims that meeting human needs requires a more humanistic approach. Furthermore, in recognising that health and illness raise fundamental existential concerns which impact on all aspects of life, the responses required of nursing need to be flexible enough to accommodate all human needs, including those of sexuality (Reimen, 1986; Benner & Wrubel, 1988).

Within this exploration of sexuality in relation to acute illness, it is proposed that three key issues require specific consideration. The first is the impact of social factors shaping healthcare cultures themselves, such as the role of nurses and their concern with body care. The second is the relationship between acute illness and sexual health and the third relates to broader questions of the impact of sexual orientation or identity within healthcare systems that may mirror general social attitudes.

Nursing work and the body

Lawler (1991) suggests that examining the relationship between nursing and the body is crucial to understanding the nature of nursing work. She quotes Turner (1984, p.1):

'In our society, the body has a fragmented, silent, and ambiguous presence despite an obvious and prominent fact about human beings: they have bodies and they are bodies... Our everyday life is dominated by details of corporeal existence, involving us in a constant labour of eating, washing, grooming, dressing and sleeping.'

Turner (1984) also suggests that nurses have daily contact with people who need help with these 'details of corporeal existence' and this involves nurses being exposed to intimate and normally private bodily activities which are expected to be managed in professional and taken-for-granted ways. This relationship between the two signifiers of the 'body as a malfunctioning machine' versus the 'body as a suffering person' has been a source of considerable debate within social theory and is certainly relevant in relation to the focus of this chapter (Kleinman, 1988). If body work in nursing requires a detached and professional approach it is clearly unrealistic to expect intimate sexual issues to be introduced with ease into such situations. This conflict of expectations may explain some of the discomfort felt when sexual concerns are manifest. Chapter 5 addresses the facets of this complex social inter-relationship between nurses, the body, body work and sexuality in more detail. Other influences such as the specific consequences of acute illness as well as social constructions of illness and illness behaviours are also worthy of consideration.

The nature of acute illness

Acute illness implies that the duration of the disease process or therapy is expected to be time-limited. Whilst some acute episodes may lead to more chronic outcomes, for example myocardial infarction may result in longer-term lifestyle changes or a need for regular follow-up, others, such as minor surgery, may involve only brief contact with healthcare services. The time available to address sexual concerns is, therefore likely to be very limited within acute care settings, reinforcing the need for accurate and appropriate methods of patient assessment, as well as access to specialist resources where necessary.

The nature of acute illness is governed by social as well as medical parameters; these parameters strongly influence how an ill person will be viewed by those with whom they come into contact. A seminal work exploring this issue was that of Parsons (1951), who introduced the concept of the 'sick role'. Parsons' work is only one of a range of sociological theories that are useful in helping to understand the importance of social influences which may shape the behaviour of someone who becomes acutely ill, as well as the professionals working with them. Parsons' theory suggests that, in order to prevent social chaos, society must exert some form of control over who is to be considered deservedly unwell. His theory proposed that the person who seeks to be considered as 'ill' must agree to fulfil certain social criteria. For example, they should withdraw from social obligations, they should be exempted responsibility for their condition, they should follow the advice of experts and seek out the best care available. When possible, they are also expected to return to their normal social role when advised to do so (Turner, 1987).

This transition from being an independent person to becoming a patient is a highly significant one that entails recognising the rules of the new role in order to justify assistance from professionals (Goffman, 1970). Passivity, compliance and deference may make it less likely that private or taboo issues, such as sexuality, are raised by a disempowered patient, even though they may be important to the life of the person.

The impact of social forces, such as the expectations of the sick role, may partly explain why sexuality has traditionally been viewed at best as a peripheral or at worst a taboo concern for acute-care settings. Figure 13.1 offers a summary of the perception of sexuality within acute care contexts.

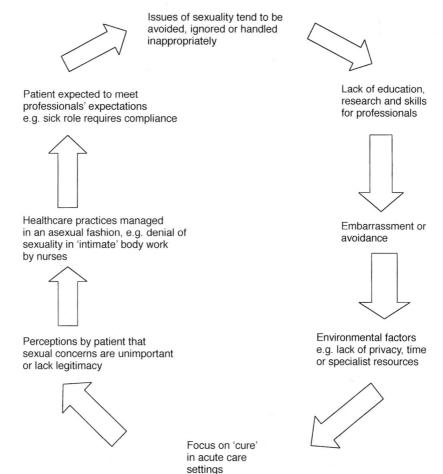

Issues of sexuality tend to be avoided, ignored or handled inappropriately

Patient expected to meet professionals' expectations e.g. sick role requires compliance

Lack of education, research and skills for professionals

Healthcare practices managed in an asexual fashion, e.g. denial of sexuality in 'intimate' body work by nurses

Embarrassment or avoidance

Perceptions by patient that sexual concerns are unimportant or lack legitimacy

Environmental factors e.g. lack of privacy, time or specialist resources

Focus on 'cure' in acute care settings

Fig. 13.1 Cyclical nature of influences that may contribute to the way sexuality is perceived in relation to acute illness.

The influence of the culture of care

The culture of the healthcare setting is constructed through the adoption of certain values, assumptions and behaviours. In relation to acute illness, the hospital culture is also shaped by set routines, professional hierarchies and unwritten rules that relay powerful messages to the patient (Schein, 1992). They signify that the main purpose of the acute setting is to cure the diseased body.

If such an environment suggests to patients that worries about sexuality are less important or less valid, they may feel disinclined to raise them. Similarly, professionals may also consider sexuality somewhat irrelevant to the purpose of the acute illness culture. They may even view sexuality as a potential threat, disrupting the management of intimate body work, for instance.

Dimensions of sexuality, power and acute illness

Definitions and clarification of terms is important in discussions such as this. Sexuality is a multidimensional concept and, in relation to acute illness, becomes relevant at several distinct levels. A useful distinction in terms to make is between 'sexual function' and 'sexual identity' in relation to the remaining focus of this chapter.

Clark (1993) defines sexual dysfunction as the inability to express one's sexuality consistent with personal needs and preferences. In health, sexual function involves the expression of sexual desires and practices that arise from highly individual perspectives.

Acute illness will obviously impact on sexual function in different ways. A patient who is in traction following a road traffic accident, for example, is likely to have little choice over how sexual function is to be expressed; furthermore, their sense of sexual satisfaction is likely to be adversely affected as a result.

The question of choice over sexual expression is relevant to a diverse range of patient populations, yet in the absence of appropriate information patients may be unable to exercise choice. For example, Jenkins (1988) found that almost 60% of women with a gynaecological malignancy received no sexual counselling either before or after treatment. If medical or surgical treatment affects an area of the body directly related to sexual function, it would appear to be only good practice to ensure that patient education related to the impact of the treatment on sexual health is provided. The reasons why this may not occur may at first be unclear until the wider questions of power, attitudes to sexuality and professional practice are considered (Fox, 1995).

The central question of power

Providing information about sexual function can be seen as an example of how deficiencies in healthcare practice may be linked with broader questions of power and control. Foucault (1976) explored the relationship between the medicalisation of the body and the consequences of this for healthcare systems. Medicine is afforded a privileged professional position and has developed its own language or 'discourses' that are closely guarded and symbolic of its expertise. As a result, the use of these discourses became powerful social tools (Fox, 1995) and any attempts to disrupt them threatened to shift the balance away from medical control towards exposing the individual or human consequences arising from disease. Authors such as Armstrong (1983) claim that, as a result, the 'ill' or 'well' body can be seen to have become a political entity in itself. Attempts to explore the personal or more private consequences of illness, such as the impact on sexuality, may challenge this dominant ideology and are likely to provoke resistance.

An example of how sexuality and power are manifested relates to how menstruation, a normal physiological occurrence, is viewed by society (Laws, 1992). In studying this topic Laws claims that menstrual disorders are viewed as '...the dirtiest of the dirty work which they [gynaecologists] must do ... menstrual problems are seen as evidence that the woman is in rebellion against, or failing at, her job of being female' (p.159).

Once again it is clear that the questions raised within this text highlight fundamental but complex issues for nurses seeking to understand the importance of human sexuality. In parallel are the moral debates, taboos and politicising processes which surround sexuality in modern culture that may explain the controversies and suspicions which this topic often evokes (Weeks, 1986). Against this complex sociopolitical background it is important to ask whether or not sexuality really is impcrtant to people when they become acutely ill.

Sexual function and acute illness

In this section some of the research which is available in relation to sexuality and acute illness will be considered and the impact of acute myocardial infarction will be explored as a key exemplar.

When exploring some of the factors that can impact on the human sexual response, Skrine (1997, p.1) states:

'Sexual activity is dependent on both physical and emotional factors. The nerves, arteries and veins to the genital organs, not to mention the hormones throughout the body, need to be working adequately. At the same time, as anyone who has ever felt the stirring of sexual arousal within themselves will know, an almost limitless expanse of emotions can enhance or subdue arousal and sexual activity.'

This statement helps to emphasise the many complex physical, social and emotional factors that can adversely affect sexual function as a result of acute illness. In the acute phase of physical illness the accompanying symptoms are likely to interfere with a person's desire for sex. Symptoms which commonly occur such as pain, fatigue, anxiety, altered elimination, breathlessness, pyrexia, light sensitivity, nausea, cramps, sweating and diminished levels of consciousness are all sufficient to diminish the human sexual response. In this acute phase the individual is likely to be focused on achieving comfort and appropriate treatment. In severe life-threatening conditions, such as myocardial infarction, the combination of pain and fear felt will cause the individual to be aware only of the need to survive this crisis and of receiving adequate help.

Sexuality and myocardial infarction

Following an event like myocardial infarction, patients will experience a number of fears about levels of exertion and how to resume normal activity safely. Masters *et al.* (1994) suggest that even during an acute illness episode, such as myocardial infarction, it is useful to remember that levels of intimacy can still be achieved, despite the absence of sexual activity itself, and are more likely to be manifest through expressions of love and concern.

Thus, whilst acutely ill people may be unable to express themselves sexually, they may still wish to engage in receiving and demonstrating reciprocal commitment and concern for those important to them. This is an interesting perspective that may help to redefine the perceived relevance of sexuality within such situations. It also stresses the importance of companionship and privacy at such times and the nurse may have a useful role in facilitating these for the patient.

It has been shown, however, that four or five days after the infarction, patients' concerns may change from those of survival to contemplating the impact of their illness on a range of issues such as work, driving or resuming sexual activity (Thompson, 1990; Piper, 1992). Although 90% of such patients may return to work, as many as 60% will continue to experience significant changes to their sexual function (Trimmer, 1986).

Acute coronary disease has attracted significant research attention, reflecting perhaps the importance of patients' fears when they have to face the return to life beyond the relative safety of the hospital. Studies by, *inter alia*, Thurer (1982), Baggs (1986), McCann (1989), Lewis and Bell (1995) and Steinke and Patterson-Midgley (1996) indicate that successful rehabilitation of such patients should include advice about, and the opportunity to explore, personal fears concerning, the safest way to resume sexual function. The availability of specialist advice is also considered a vital component of rehabilitation for such patients. An interesting point to note, however, is that few studies have yet investigated the specific sexual rehabilitation needs of women after myocardial infarction (Baggs & Karch, 1987).

In terms of providing specific educational interventions for patients recovering from myocardial infarction, there are a number of resources now available. For example, Albarran and Bridger (1997) describe the development of an information leaflet to answer patients' questions about resuming their sex lives, adopting a conversational style with minimal use of medical jargon. The content of this written educational material was based upon questions a patient or partner might ask as highlighted in previous research studies and included issues such as the following.

- When is it OK to start making love again?
- Does sexual intercourse put a strain on the heart?
- I don't feel like making love anymore.
- My partner doesn't seem very keen to make love.
- Which position is the safest?
- What should I do if I get chest pain during sex?
- Could the tablets I am taking affect my sex life?
- Should I ever avoid sexual intercourse?

(Albarran & Bridger, 1997)

It is known that the severity of the infarction is a less significant factor in sexual debility than the psychological state of the patient (Thompson, 1990). Thus, a patient who is worryied about resuming sexual activity may benefit significantly from access to written information to reinforce the verbal advice previously provided. Practical strategies may be preferred by patients (Turton, 1998) and include, for example, advice on the use of sub-lingual nitrates prior to sexual activity to prevent angina pain, or the avoidance of anal intercourse during the recovery period to avoid vagal stimulation (Seidle *et al.*, 1991).

Myocardial infarction is an example of an acute illness episode that can clearly impact on all aspects of an individual's life, including their sexual expression. Considerable attention has been focused on understanding the rehabilitation needs of these patients, including the resumption of sexual expression as an integral part of the rehabilitation process.

Sexuality and research into other acute conditions

Surgery

Surgery can alter the body dramatically and may lead to considerable anxiety about re-establishing satisfactory sexual relationships. Studies by Gloeckner (1984), Cohen *et al.* (1989), Bohachick *et al.* (1992), Kaplan (1992) and Lamb and Sheldon (1994) support this assertion; their findings indicate that patients frequently need help in addressing sexual and relationship concerns, and that nurses have an important role to play in encouraging discussion of these as part of the care package.

Drug therapy

Drug therapy used in acute illness is also an important factor to consider as this may significantly impact on normal sexual function. Examples of drugs that may be especially important include cytotoxic chemotherapy agents (Auchincloss, 1989), hormonal agents, anti-hypertensives, beta blockers, diuretics, sedatives, opioids and amphetamines (Tomlinson, 1999). Drug therapy is a common treatment for most acute illnesses and patients may only notice significant alterations in their sexual interest or satisfaction after some time. A useful strategy may be to provide written information that includes an explanation of the sexual side effects of medication as well as indicating further sources of help or advice. Perhaps one of the main challenges is to increase the level of awareness among professionals themselves about this issue.

Sexual health experiences of other patient groups

People who have experienced sudden traumatic injury have been the focus of considerable research in relation to recovery of sexual function. Focusing on spinal cord injury, for example, studies have identified common experiences such as having to adapt to new forms of sexual expression instead of intercourse. The need for appropriate interventions such as structured sexual counselling or specially designed sexual education programmes have also been highlighted from such research (Kennedy & Over, 1990; Pilsecker, 1990; Sipski & Alexander, 1993; Kreuter *et al.*, 1996).

It is interesting to note that other patient groups who have experienced sexual difficulties have generally attracted less attention within the literature, although some additional examples are worth noting. For instance, there are studies focusing on the sexual health impact of a diverse range of medical conditions including cerebrovascular accident (Burgener & Logan, 1989), renal failure

(Milde *et al.*, 1996), inflammatory bowel disease (Giese & 1996), skin disorders (Buckwater, 1982), diabetes (LeMone, ⅃ joint replacement surgery (Spica & Schwab, 1996), epilepsy (Mims, 1996), rheumatic disease (Dale, 1996) and low back pain (Ritchie & Daines, 1992).

Whilst the available research helps to identify sexual concerns that patients with specific conditions may have, a common theme which emerges from them all is that sexual function is a relevant concern in acute illness. Patients do want this issue to be addressed by a suitably skilled person and at an appropriate time. It also has to be stressed that there remains enormous scope for further research with patient groups whose needs may currently be unknown.

An example of how failing to address sexual functioning can have significant impact on the individual was highlighted to me during the course of a research project into the needs of men with prostate cancer. One man, speaking of how the diagnosis was made following a transrectal ultrasound and prostatic biopsy, said: 'No one told me my ejaculate would come out bloody. I really thought I was dead...'. This indicates once again that even when there are clear links between sexual function and the site of a suspected malignancy, no mention of what to expect had been offered to help this man. His shock was obvious in the research interview even though the incident had taken place some years before.

Strategies for encouraging awareness of sexual health needs in acute settings

In order to ensure that the sexual health needs of patients are identified, two main strategies are essential. The first is to stress the importance of comprehensive patient assessment using a relevant framework and documentation of need (Kelly *et al.*, 1996). By assessing individuals' level of knowledge about their illness, and the possible consequences of proposed treatments, concerns around sexual issues may be covered in a sensitive and appropriate manner. Waxman (1993), whilst exploring assessment of sexual concerns within the context of cancer care, suggests that simple questions such as 'Has cancer changed the way you see yourself as a man?' can help to highlight pertinent concerns and give the individual permission to disclose as much as they wish.

Skrine (1997) also reinforces the need to listen, to give advice if appropriate, to use reassurance sparingly and to learn to tolerate the feeling of sometimes not knowing what to do or say in such situations.

The P-LI-SS-IT model (Annon, 1976) is also a useful example of a counselling tool that may be useful for nurses in busy clinical settings. The P-LI-SS-IT acronym which stands for Permission, Limited Information, Specific Suggestions, and Intensive Therapy is discussed in more detail in Chapter 16 and reinforces the important first step of allowing the issue of sexuality to be voiced.

Champion (1996) has proposed use of the ALARM model, as it provides a clear structure against which sexual function can be assessed, for example:

Activity (such as normal level of interest in sex, modes of sexual expression, form of sexual relationships)
Libido (any changes from normal pattern, how important is this, is the person satisfied with current situation?)
Arousal (are there any specific problems such as difficulties in achieving or maintaining erection or vaginal lubrication; does this lead to emotional or relationship disruption?)
Resolution (is the level of orgasm satisfying; are there any problems with pain or discomfort?)
Medical history (are there any underlying physical or emotional causes which need to be explored, is the person currently taking medication or recovering from illness?).

This format for approaching sexual assessment may be of practical use in busy settings and provides a structure within which sensitive questions can be phrased.

The second strategy that requires attention is how to encourage nurses to actually address sexuality within the reality of demanding clinical roles and against a background of limited education or training. It is unrealistic to assume that an easy solution exists when important barriers such as personal attitudes and prejudices, lack of knowledge and privacy require attention and action (Gamel *et al.*, 1993). Recent attempts to confront these difficulties have been emerging in the literature but it would appear that a more concerted effort is necessary to ensure that all healthcare professionals are better prepared to address sexual health needs within their practice (Van Ooijen & Charnock, 1994; Dennison, 1997).

A review of selected research on barriers to integration of sexuality within nursing practice, together with suggested strategies to overcome them, is discussed further in Chapter 16.

The importance of sexual identity and the acute illness experience

The final issue to be addressed in relation to acute illness concerns sexual orientation or identity. The work of Kinsey *et al.* (1948, 1953), which first described the continuum of human sexuality, were highly influential publications of their time, and suggested that homosexuality and heterosexuality were not necessarily exclusive propositions for many people. Those whose sexual identity differs from the espoused heterosexual norm, however, still commonly experience discrimination and prejudice. The issue of provision of non-prejudicial care is also addressed in Chapters 4 and 16.

Sexuality has been described as:

'...the most natural thing about us. It is the basis for some of our most passionate feelings and commitments. Through it we experience ourselves as real people; it gives us our identities, our sense of self, as men and women, as heterosexual and homosexual, "normal" or "abnormal", "natural" or "unnatural".'

(Weeks, 1986, p.13)

Research has indicated that there are often negative attitudes displayed towards certain patient groups, especially those who are gay or lesbian (Douglas *et al.*, 1985; Young, 1988; Akinsanya & Rouse, 1992; James *et al.*, 1994). In the study by James *et al.* (1994) negative attitudes had been displayed in various ways towards lesbian or gay patients. These included patients feeling ignored; being seen as sexually threatening to staff; feeling that staff were unwilling to initiate discussions about sexual issues; experiencing insensitive interviewing and being pressurised into agreeing to certain treatments.

It is important to stress that acute illness will normally involve fear and anxiety anyway and attitudes such as those exposed in the studies mentioned above indicate some of the extra pressures which acutely ill gay patients may also have to cope with.

An incident related to the author, by a young gay man, also illustrates this additional psychological burden. When preparing to undergo a serious cardiac operation, the most worrying thing to him was being anaesthetised in case he disclosed something about his sexuality and 'word would get out'. This burden was being carried over and above his anxieties about his surgery. Staff would perhaps never know what was really troubling him because no one would actually ask.

Conclusion

This chapter has focused on the importance of sexuality in acute illness and suggests that this issue is best understood from three distinct dimensions. The first dimension involves the influence of sexuality in relation to the culture of acute health care and on the roles of both patient and nurse. The second dimension concerns the impact that illness and treatment can have on sexual expression and thus sexual health itself and the third dimension relates to the importance of recognising negative attitudes to patients whose

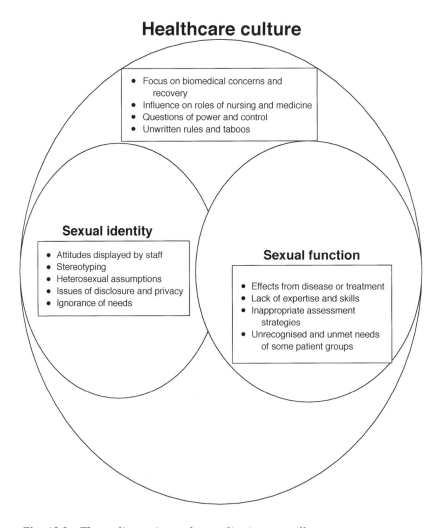

Healthcare culture

- Focus on biomedical concerns and recovery
- Influence on roles of nursing and medicine
- Questions of power and control
- Unwritten rules and taboos

Sexual identity

- Attitudes displayed by staff
- Stereotyping
- Heterosexual assumptions
- Issues of disclosure and privacy
- Ignorance of needs

Sexual function

- Effects from disease or treatment
- Lack of expertise and skills
- Inappropriate assessment strategies
- Unrecognised and unmet needs of some patient groups

Fig. 13.2 Three dimensions of sexuality in acute illness.

sexual preferences may differ from our own. The relationships between these various dimensions are represented in Fig. 13.2.

From the published work available it is clear that sexuality is a legitimate issue worthy of further research within acute care and nurses do have a significant contribution to make within both sexuality research and practice development. In terms of acute illness less time may be available to negotiate what is important to the patient in terms of their intimate relationships. This fact alone makes awareness of sexuality in such settings even more relevant. The evidence about the sexual rehabilitation needs of patients experiencing myocardial infarction demonstrates that it is possible to translate research findings into practical interventions such as patient-friendly information resources.

As stated from the outset, effective health care in acute care settings involves seeing beyond a disease or condition to an individual with unique needs. The issues surrounding human sexuality demonstrate just how challenging it can be to realise this in practice. Through being aware of how powerfully sexuality impacts on the culture of acute health care, as well as appreciating its relevance to holistic practice, we are provided with considerable scope for research, education and practice development for the future.

References

Akinsanya, J. & Rouse, P. (1992) Who will care? A survey of the knowledge and attitudes of hospital nurses to people with HIV/AIDS. *Journal of Advanced Nursing*, **17**, 3, 400–401.

Albarran, J. & Bridger, S. (1997) Problems with providing education on resuming sexual activity after myocardial infarction: developing written information for patients. *Intensive and Critical Care Nursing*, **13**, 2–11.

Annon, J.S. (1976) The P-LI-SS-IT Model: A proposed conceptual scheme for the behavioural treatment of sexual problems. *Journal of Sex Education and Therapy*, **2**, 2, 1–15.

Armstrong, D. (1983) *Political Anatomy of the Body*. Cambridge University Press, Cambridge.

Armstrong, D. (1987) Theoretical tensions in biopsychosocial medicine. *Social Science and Medicine*, **25**, 11, 1213–18.

Auchincloss, S.S. (1989) Sexual dysfunction in cancer patients: issues in evaluation and treatment. In: J. Holland & C. Rowland (eds) *Handbook of Psycho-Oncology: Psychological Care of the Patient with Cancer*. Oxford University Press, New York.

Baggs, J. (1986) Nursing diagnosis: potential sexual dysfunction after myocardial infarction. *Dimensions of Critical Care Nursing*, **13**, 1, 2–11.

Baggs, J.G. & Karch, A.M. (1987) Sexual counselling of women with coronary heart disease. *Heart and Lung*, **16**, 2, 154–9.

Benner, P. & Wrubel, J. (1988) *The Primacy of Caring*. Addison-Wesley, San Francisco.

Bohachick, P., Anton, B.B., Wooldridge, P.J., Kormos, R.L., Armitage, J.M., Hardesty, R.L. & Griffin, B.P. (1992) Psychosocial outcome six months after heart transplant surgery: a preliminary report. *Research in Nursing and Health*, **15**, 3, 165–73.

Buckwater, K.C. (1982) The influence of skin conditions on sexual expression. *Sexuality and Disability*, **5**, 2, 98–106.

Burgener, S. & Logan, G. (1989) Sexuality concerns of the post-stroke patient. *Rehabilitation Nursing*, **14**, 4, 178–81.

Champion, A. (1996) Male cancer and sexual function. *Sexual and Marital Therapy*, **11**, 3, 227–44.

Clark, J. (1993) Psychosocial responses of the patient: altered sexual health. In: S.I. Groenwald, M.H. Frogge, M. Goodman & C.H. Yarbro (eds) *Cancer Nursing Principles and Practice*. Jones & Bartlett, London.

Cohen, S.M., Hollingsworth, A.O. & Rubin, M. (1989) Another look at psychologic complications of hysterectomy. *Image*, **21**, 1, 51–3.

Dale, K.G. (1996) Intimacy and rheumatic disease. *Rehabilitation Nursing*, **21**, 1, 38–40.

Dennison, S. (1997) Psycho-sexual care for patients with cancer and their partners: a service development. *Journal of Cancer Nursing*, **1**, 3, 141–3.

Douglas, C.J., Kalman, C.M. & Kalman, T.P. (1985) Homophobia among physicians and nurses: an empirical study. *Hospital and Community Psychiatry*, **36**, 12, 1309–11.

Elston, M.A. (1991) The politics of professional power: medicine in a changing health service In: J. Gabe, M. Calnan & M. Bury (eds) *Sociology of the Health Service*. Routledge, London.

Foucault, M. (1976) *The Birth of the Clinic*. Tavistock, London.

Fox, N. (1995) *Postmodernism, Sociology and Health*. Open University Press, Buckingham.

Gamel, C., Davis, B.D. & Hengeveld, M. (1993) Nurses' provision of teaching and counselling on sexuality: a review of the literature. *Journal of Advanced Nursing*, **18**, 8, 1219–27.

Giese, L.A. & Terrell, L. (1996) Sexual health issues in inflammatory bowel disease. *Gastroenterology Nursing*, **19**, 1, 12–17.

Gloeckner, M.R. (1984) Perceptions of sexual attractiveness following ostomy surgery. *Research in Nursing and Health*, **7**, 2, 87–92.

Goffman, E. (1970) *Stigma: Notes on the Management of Spoiled Identity*. Penguin Books, Harmondsworth.

James, T., Harding, I. & Corbett, K. (1994) Biased care? *Nursing Times*, **90**, 51, 28–30.

Jenkins, B. (1988) Reports of sexual changes after treatment for gynaecological cancer. *Oncology Nursing Forum*, **15**, 3, 349–54.

Kaplan, H.S. (1992) A neglected issue: the sexual side effects of current treatments for breast cancer. *Journal of Sexual and Marital Therapy*, **18**, 1, 3–9.

Kelly, D., Scott, K. & Speechley, V. (1996) Assessment, communication and consent. In: J. Mallett & C. Bailey (eds) *The Royal Marsden Hospital Manual of Clinical Nursing Procedures*. Blackwell Science, London.

Kennedy, S. & Over, R. (1990) Psychophysiological assessment of male sexual function following spinal cord injury. *Archives of Sexual Behaviour*, **19**, 1, 15–27.

Kinsey, A.C., Pomeroy, W.B., Martin, C.E. & Gebhard, P.H. (1948) *Sexual Behaviour in the Human Male*. WB Saunders, Philadelphia.

Kinsey, A.C., Pomeroy, W.B., Martin, C.E. & Gebhard, P.H. (1953) *Sexual Behaviour in the Human Female*. WB Saunders, Philadelphia.

Kleinman, A. (1988) *The Illness Narratives*. Basic Books, New York.

Kreuter, M., Sullivan, M. & Siosteen, A. (1996) Sexual adjustment after spinal cord injury – comparisons of partner experiences in pre- and post-injury relationships. *Paraplegia*, **32**, 11, 759–70.

Lamb, M.A. & Sheldon, T.A. (1994) The sexual adaptation of women treated for endometrial cancer. *Cancer* Practice, **2**, 2, 103–13.

Lawler, J. (1991) *Behind the Screens: Nursing, Somology and the Problem of the Body*. Churchill Livingstone, Edinburgh.

Laws, S. (1992) *Issues of Blood: The Politics of Menstruation*. Macmillan, London.

LeMone, P. (1996) The physical effects of diabetes on sexuality in women. *Diabetes Education*, **22**, 4, 361–6.

Lewis, D. & Bell, S.K. (1995) Pulmonary rehabilitation, psychosocial adjustment and use of healthcare services. *Rehabilitation Nursing*, **20**, 2, 102–7.

Masters, W.H., Johnson, V.E. & Kolodny, R.C. (1994) *Heterosexuality*. Harper Collins, London.

McCann, M.E. (1989) Sexual healing after heart attack. *American Journal of Nursing*, **89**, 9, 1132–8.

Milde, F.K., Hart, L.K. & Fearing, M.O. (1996) Sexuality and fertility concerns of dialysis patients. *Annals of the North American Nurses Association*, **23**, 3, 307–15.

Mims, J. (1996) Sexuality and related issues in the preadolescent and adolescent female with epilepsy. *Journal of Neuroscience Nursing*, **28**, 2, 102–6.

Parsons, T. (1951) *The Social System*. Free Press, Illinois.

Pilsecker, C. (1990) Starting out: the first 6 months post hospital for spinal cord-injured veterans. *American Journal of Physical Medicine*, **69**, 2, 91–5.

Piper, K.M. (1992) When can I do it again? Sexual counselling after a heart attack. *Professional Nurse*, **8**, 3, 168–72.

Reimen, D. (1986) Noncaring and caring in the clinical setting: patients' descriptions. *Topics in Clinical Nursing*, **8**, 2, 30–36.

Ritchie, M.H. & Daines, B. (1992) Sexuality and low back pain. *British Journal of Occupational Therapy*, **55**, 9, 347–50.

Schein, E. (1992) *Organisational Culture and Leadership*. Jossey-Bass, San Francisco.

Seidle, A., Bullough, B., Haughey, B., Scherer, Y., Rhodes, M. & Brown, G. (1991) Understanding the effects of a myocardial infarction on sexual functioning: A basis for sexual counselling. *Rehabilitation Nurse*, **16**, 255–64.

Sipski, M.L. & Alexander, C.J. (1993) Sexual activities, response and satisfaction in women pre- and post-spinal cord injury. *Archives of Physical Medicine and Rehabilitation*, **74**, 10, 1025–9.

Skrine, R. (1997) *Blocks and Freedoms in Sexual Life*. Radcliffe Medical Press, Oxford.

Spica, M.M. & Schwab, M.D. (1996) Sexual expression after total joint replacement. *Orthopaedic Nursing*, **15**, 5, 41–4.

Steinke, E. & Patterson-Midgley, P. (1996) Sexual counselling following acute myocardial infarction. *Clinical Nursing Research*, **5**, 4, 462–72.

Thompson, D. (1990) The coronary patient and his spouse. *Nursing*, **4**, 3, 6–8.

Thurer, S.L. (1982) The long-term sexual response to coronary bypass surgery: some preliminary findings. *Sexuality and Disability*, **5**, 4, 208–12.

Tomlinson, J. (1999) Taking a sexual history. In: *The ABC of Sexual Health*. British Medical Journal (BMJ) Publications, London.

Trimmer, E. (1986) Is it safe to have sex following heart disease? *Midwife, Health Visitor and Community Nurse*, **22**, 10, 344.

Turner, B.S. (1984) *The Body and Society: Explorations in Social Theory*. Basil Blackwell, Oxford.

Turner, B.S. (1987) *Medical Power and Social Knowledge*. Sage Publications, London.

Turton, J. (1998) Importance of information following myocardial infarction: a study of the self-perceived information of patients and their spouse/partner compared with the perceptions of nursing staff. *Journal of Advanced Nursing*, **27**, 770–78.

Van Ooijen, E.V. & Charnock, A. (1994) *Sexuality and Patient Care: A Guide for Nurses and Teachers*. Chapman & Hall, London.

Waxman, E.S. (1993) Sexual dysfunction following treatment for prostate cancer: nursing assessment and interventions. *Oncology Nursing Forum*, **20**, 10, 1567–71.

Weeks, J. (1986) *Sexuality*. Tavistock Publications, London.

Young, E.W. (1988) Nurses' attitudes towards homosexuality. *Journal of Continuing Education in Nursing*, **19**, 1, 9–12.

14. *Sexuality and People with Disability or Chronic Illness*

Carole Webster and Hazel Heath

Society is trying hard to accommodate its disabled and chronically ill population. Ramps have been constructed for new buildings, toilet facilities have been provided in shopping centres and restaurants. Employers are finally starting to recognise that people with disabilities can be productive and an asset to their business and educational mainstreaming is in progress. Since the early 1980s, the openness of well-known celebrities has enhanced awareness of the realities of living with chronic illness, and writings by disabled people have transformed our understanding of the real nature of disability from that of a medical model to that of a social one (Oliver, 1990). But what about sexuality? Somehow western culture cannot associate being disabled or chronically ill with being sexual, for example, until recently, 'sexuality' and 'disability' were words which rarely appeared together (Morgan, 1994).

This chapter aims to explore key issues facing people with disability or chronic illness in expressing sexuality. It highlights societal attitudes and how these might impact on individuals. It identifies some realities faced by people with disability or chronic illness and how health professionals can help, particularly in the maintenance of individual identities and choices in living. While the chapter largely discusses disability, this term aims to encompass consideration of the disabling effects of chronic illness, for example the tremor of Parkinson's disease or multiple sclerosis; the breathlessness of pulmonary disease or cardiac failure, or the restricted mobility and joint swelling associated with arthritis. This chapter also acknowledges the impact of less obvious symptoms such as chronic fatigue or pain, which can be equally disabling.

The diversity of causes and effects of disability and chronic illness is immense and each person's experience is unique, yet there is a tendency for people, including those with signs of chronic illness, to be lumped into a homogenous entity and labelled as 'disabled' (Cooper & Guillebaud, 1999). There may be similarities between the issues faced by individuals, but essentially each person is unique as are their wishes, aspirations, and the realities of the experiences in their everyday lives.

Disability – definitions, images and attitudes

Attitudes to disability are manifest in many ways, ranging from non-acknowledgement and negative images to overt discrimination. Until relatively recently, people with disabilities were omitted from consideration within many key national and local policies which impact upon them. Disability is reinforced through 'non-ready' access, reduced opportunities or discrimination, and individual citizens can be as disadvantaged by unemployment, poverty, inaccessible public transport and prejudice as they are by their physical limitations (Cooper & Guillebaud, 1999). 'Disabled people want to see removal of barriers to leading full and active lives, not changes in their physical difference.' (Shakespeare *et al.*, 1996, p.184)

People's freedom to express themselves as sexual beings, to engage in relationships and to be sexually active is potentially disabled by the images and attitudes that surround them. Images of disabled people looking 'sexy' or engaging in sexual activities are rarely seen. *Playboy* magazine once featured a centrefold of a disabled woman but her legs were covered and she did not pose in her wheelchair. There are disabled models but they mainly feature in advertisements for disability-related products and rarely, if ever, in mainstream advertising. Conversely, able-bodied models appear in adverts for products designed for people with disabilities or chronic illness.

Until relatively recently, films and television programmes were worse in their denial of the sexual identity of people with a disability. *Born on the Fourth of July* and *Coming Home* depicted paralysed men sexually satisfying women. Several soaps have characters with disabilities, for example *Emmerdale*'s Chris Tate and *Coronation Street*'s Jim McDonald, both addressing the issue of sexuality but interestingly neither actor is disabled. The film *The Theory of Flight* promised to be the most important and moving film in recent years about disability. The actress who portrayed a disabled woman said that she felt a fraud while working with disabled extras during the filming. In 1998, Equity, the actors' union, changed its rules to ensure that disabled actors were always given first consideration in the portrayal of people with disabilities.

Brown *et al.* (2000) suggest that societal views on sexuality and disability can be summarised by four stances.

- *The ostrich position:* you must be joking – sex isn't for the likes of you.
- *Only beautiful people need apply:* this is our scene and you have to be young, fit and thin before we let you in.
- *The sex aids and implants approach:* this should help you to perform as if you were normal, here are some sex aids.
- *Proud visibility:* you set the agenda. We will help you in so far as you want us to. We recognise your right to find your own way and celebrate your sexuality in proud and maybe even shocking ways.

While these approaches can be acknowledged at a societal level, issues within different societal groups and sub-cultures are very distinct. For example, both gender and ethnicity distinctions have been identified in terms of employment and income status for people with disabilities (Pfeiffer, 1991).

Hanna and Rogovsky (1991) found that compared with disabled men, disabled women were less likely to be well educated, in well-paid employment or to stay married. Distinctions in expectations have also been identified, for example Shakespeare *et al.* (1996, p.96) suggested that disabled men are encouraged to be 'superman' while disabled females may be discounted as women by expectations to be 'beautiful' or through ill-informed perceptions related to the advisability of bearing children. Brown *et al.* (2000, p.44) also identify a potential for abuse by 'a certain type of man [who] gravitates towards disabled women'. This, they suggest, is not so much about an intimate relationship as an issue of power and control.

Disabled people from black and ethnic minority groups not only have to contend with the disablement which western society enforces through lack of access, employment and other resources, but additionally in relation to a predominantly white disability movement and prejudices within their own communities (Brown *et al.*, 2000). For example, there may be cultural expectations and customs around personal hygiene, skin care, gender and caring roles (Bignall & Butt, 1999) which can particularly impact on individuals who need help with personal care. One member of the core group in Brown *et al.*'s project (2000, p.48) described how she had

213

defied her own community and its religious teachings in deciding not to marry or have children because she was disabled. Strong cultural sanctions may also exist for same gender relationships.

The realities of living with disability or chronic illness

Disabilities may be congenital or become apparent during childhood. Disabled children from a range of cultures have expressed frustration about being overprotected and not afforded the same freedoms to develop social relationships as their peers who do not have disabilities. This can be particularly difficult during adolescence when the need to establish identity and explore relationships can become acute (Morris, 1999; Bignall & Butt, 2000). Disability arising in adulthood may herald multiple changes in life affecting independence, freedom to move around, employment and changes in the balance of relationships, particularly with a partner. At first sight, the loss of sexual fulfilment may seem a minor consequence of disability or the onset of chronic illness when set against the profound effects of the changes on all aspects of life. Nevertheless, sexuality can link fundamentally with self-esteem and, as Kellett (1990) highlights, when a healthy active man or woman is turned into a 'cripple' overnight the retention of self-esteem is essential.

Adults who acquire a severe disability, for example paralysis following an accident, ideally have structured rehabilitation programmes where attention is paid to the need for rebuilding sexuality expression in the context of newly constructed lives. However, many people who develop disabilities suddenly, for example through a cerebrovascular accident or back injury, are not offered adequate rehabilitation. Many other people develop disabilities gradually, for example through arthritis, chronic obstructive pulmonary disease or multiple sclerosis. Where do they turn for help and advice?

Chronic illnesses are lifelong and entail lifetime adaptations but the 'trajectories' of chronic diseases and disabilities vary greatly. Corbin and Strauss (1988) suggest there are several discernible phases in chronic illness, namely preventative, definitive, crisis, acute, comeback, stable, unstable, deterioration and death. Movement through the phases may be upward, downward or across a plateau and the precise trajectory varies with the individual and the disorder. The illness may progress slowly, relentlessly or unpredictably through exacerbation and remissions or the superimposition of other disorders. Treatments may change the projected course of the disability and the work involved in managing an illness at different phases in the trajectory will vary enormously (Strauss *et al.*, 1984).

For example, the initial vague symptoms of multiple sclerosis or Parkinson's disease, the remissions and relapses and the unpredictable nature of the illness can lead to distress and fear of what the future may hold. Peace (1996) describes the many losses to which people with chronic illness must adjust: decreased mobility and energy levels can be devastating, involving loss of employment, social contact and ability to care for oneself. When a chronic condition becomes part of everyday life, relationships are deeply affected and any form of social (and thus sexual) life becomes increasingly difficult as a result of fatigue, reduced mobility and finances. Changes in sexual functioning can be insidious but no less devastating than other changes.

Disabling conditions inevitably impact upon sexuality (Rieve, 1989). The inability, real or perceived, to perform sexually in the same manner as before may become a stumbling block to relationship happiness as well as to a healthy ego. Feelings of self-worth and attractiveness are threatened at a time when need for intimacy and belonging is greatest, often causing a sense of loneliness and isolation (Glass & Padrone, 1978). Those who feel sexually unattractive often tend to feel sexually worthless.

The loss of body parts can have profound psychological consequences, giving rise to grief for loss of body image, function or both. Anxiety, depression and sexual problems are related to the magnitude and type of loss as well as the personal vulnerability of the patient (Maguire, 1989; Parkes, 1991). There are few comparative studies but the effects of such losses on sexuality, across diagnostic groups, are surprisingly similar (Fallowfield *et al.*, 1986; Maguire, 1989; Hannah *et al.*, 1992; Nissen & Newman, 1992; Schag, 1994; Borowicz *et al.*, 1996).

Despite the widespread nature of sexual problems in people with disabilities and chronic illness, these are detected and treated in only a minority of patients. Clinical psychologists have much to offer in challenging patients' misconceptions of themselves and can be helpful where body image problems persist.

Two problems commonly experienced by people with disabilities or chronic illness are those of fatigue and pain. The impact of these is often underestimated and they are offered here as clinical exemplars.

Fatigue

Chronic fatigue syndrome or myalgic encephalomyelitis (ME) is estimated to affect 1–2% of the population (Royal College of

Physicians, 1996) but fatigue occurs with any disabling condition and, particularly when associated with pain, can leave the patient exhausted both physically and emotionally. Individuals have fluctuating internal and external resources, including motivation and physical or emotional strength, but energy can be drained by even straightforward activities. Helen Scott (cited in Cohen, 1997) recalled '...on a bad day I just get up, dress myself and cope with the basics. On a good day I will do light chores in the house and walk up and down the garden.' Finding energy for sexual activity can be challenging. To be able to lead anything like a normal life can take considerable planning and the need to avoid fatigue can then take over life. The reality of the fatigue experienced by many people living with chronic disorders is seldom considered in its full significance (Turner & Hughes, 1999).

Pain

It is estimated that chronic pain affects 11% of the UK population (Potter, 1989) and that approximately three-quarters of chronic pain sufferers experience some form of sexual dysfunction, yet little has been written about sex and chronic pain. For people who live with chronic pain, sexual expression often becomes disrupted and inhibited. Fearful of aggravating or exacerbating the pain, individuals are often reluctant to engage in sexual activity and many resort to total abstinence.

Offering sensitive advice

As discussed elsewhere in this book, the discomfort felt by health and social care professionals when discussing anything related to sexuality may result in the offering of vague platitudes and reassurances as opposed to the specific practical advice many people with a disability or chronic illness seek. The following guidance was written by a disabled person experiencing chronic pain (Webster, 1997) and may help healthcare professionals to consider the quality of information related to sexuality they give to their patients.

(1) Be totally honest with your partner, most partners are afraid of having any physical contact with the person experiencing pain for fear of hurting them. Do explain what hurts and what does not, where they can touch and where not and just how much pressure to apply, for example some pain is activated by a light touch, others much deeper.

216

(2)   If you are the person in pain, honesty extends to telling your partner that you feel you want sexual contact or intercourse, and this may be difficult if you are not usually the initiator of the contact. I remember one patient was most upset when she felt that her partner was ignoring her when she felt like intercourse some months after surgery. As I explained to her, he had no way of knowing this if she did not tell him how she was feeling.

(3)   Most people think of sexual contact occurring at bedtime, but chronic pain does lead to fatigue and many people in chronic pain only want a mug of cocoa at the end of the day, not sexual activity. Work out when your pain is at its lowest level; could this be the time for sexual activity? There is no rule book indicating that afternoons cannot be used. This can be difficult if you have small children around but the problem can be overcome with planning.

(4)   Do time your medication in order that it is having most effect when you make love. There is no reason why TENS machines cannot be used whilst love making, but do be aware that with movement you could have an increase or decrease of stimulation from the electrodes. They may also be pulled off if the leads are not adjusted.

(5)   Depending on the type of pain and disability the 'traditional' positions for intercourse may be impossible to use, but there are many others that can accommodate most physical problems. The organisation SPOD (the Association to Aid the Sexual and Personal Relationships of People with a Disability) have an excellent series of leaflets which discuss different positions, aids and other advice that includes a counselling service.

(6)   Many people experience a loss of libido and sometimes men fail to achieve an erection as a result of the pain and fatigue they experience, and many drugs do have a significant effect on libido. Although it may be difficult for you, do not hesitate to discuss these problems with your doctor. Often switching to another drug may help. Intercourse may be difficult due to a reduction in vaginal secretions but there are many vaginal lubricants on the market that will overcome this problem, possibly the most readily available of which is KY Jelly®. However, do not always assume your pain is the cause of problems; are you near the menopause? Again, do not be afraid to discuss this with your doctor.

(7)   If achieving or sustaining an erection is a problem, there are

217

many aids available to assist with this problem. SPOD can provide details of those available but again do discuss this with your doctor.

(8) Most people think about intercourse when sexual relations are concerned. If intercourse is not possible there are many ways to have a full and meaningful relationship without it. Many patients will describe finding other parts of their body which when caressed by a loving partner can give great fulfilment. Touch is so very important.

(9) Another taboo subject is that of masturbation, and yet this is an excellent way to explore your own body and find areas that give pleasure. Also experimenting with the differing positions suggested for intercourse may give you the confidence to try them out with a partner. Remember hurt does not always mean harm and relaxation does help pain. Why not use masturbation as a technique to give your partner pleasure if full intercourse is not possible.

(10) There are many resources available; SPOD has already been mentioned but also the Internet has a variety of web sites that deal openly and sensitively with this subject. If you use your search engine, type in disability and sexuality and not only will you find information about resources but also a chance to read about other peoples' experiences.

Changing relationships – issues for partners

The impact of disability or chronic illness on partners should never be underestimated. Partners can find themselves in totally new situations. They have to deal with the changes in their partner and to try to support their partner in coping with these, as well as with the changes in the nature of their relationship. They may feel that the needs of the person experiencing the illness or disability are paramount and therefore their own needs must be secondary. Concerns may not be verbalised or even confronted and can fester. Avoidance of making sexual demands, by either partner, can lead not only to frustration but can feel like rejection. In no longer being a sexual partner and no longer feeling desirable or attractive, the disabled person thus has their negative view of themselves reinforced (Cooper & Guillebaud, 1999).

Partners can also find themselves taking on new roles and these can have considerable impact on an intimate and sexual relationship. Take, for example, the impact of urinary incontinence on partners. Roe and May's (1999) interviewees commented that having to undertake personal care had a detrimental effect on their relationships and that incontinence could even end sexual attraction. The act of cleaning and washing the affected partner to remove urine and sometimes faeces was, in one husband's words, 'a passion killer'. Parker (1993) highlighted that female carers found it difficult to undertake personal tasks for their partners because they were aware of the partner's discomfort in being helped. Sherman (1998) suggests that there are spouses who manage to cope well with an incontinent partner but that others feel duty bound by their marriage vows to give physical caring and to meet sexual needs. Some spouses said that, despite their partner's incontinence, they would not move out of the marital bed, even if this meant changing the sheets several times a night. Some also said that they would never contemplate rebuffing the partner's sexual advances, even though they no longer gained any pleasure from sex. However, this latter stance begs the question what impact does such 'sensitivity' have on the emotional closeness and sexual satisfaction for each individual within such a relationship?

Individual identities

Self-concept, identity and self-esteem are essential to humans and certainly to the expression of sexuality. Disability and chronic illness can fundamentally challenge these in ways that can be extremely difficult to deal with. The following quotes illustrate some of the difficulties in striking a balance between realities and aspirations or between fighting and accepting help. Ultimately, even determining which aspects of one's identities to express to others necessitates striking a balance.

Some feminist writers contend that if disabled women hide their vulnerability, and gloss over the negative impact of impairment, this colludes with oppression rather than challenging it (Morris, 1991). Another said:

> 'By denying the realities of our lives, which are sometimes painful and sad, we are just swapping the "tragic and brave" model the world is so fond of for another kind of dangerous myth in which we must always be fighters.'
>
> (Keith, 1994, p.7)

A third made a plea not to be labelled as 'special needs'. 'Disabled people have the same needs as non-disabled people: the only difference is that disabled people's needs are not met'

(Heather Frances, a black disabled activist, cited in Brown *et al.*, 2000, p.23).

Ultimately, how each person constructs and chooses to assert his or her identity must be determined by individual choice: 'Disabled people enter relationships out of the strengths of their own identities as persons with disabilities' (Longmore, 1987, p.73). However, identities, and the expression of varying aspects of them, are complex. This is highlighted in Appleby's (1994) work where disabled lesbian women chose to express publicly some aspects of their identities, while keeping others private. One woman did not wish to come out as a lesbian because she feared the aggression that might attract and felt unable to defend herself because of her disabilities. She said (p.24):

> 'Of course I see myself first and foremost as a woman. My social status and sexuality and my disability are all part and parcel of who I am. I want people to be aware of that and take it on board, the whole person, and not just the bits they want.'

Another found it easier to come out as a lesbian before she did as a disabled person. She felt this had a lot to do with the fact that society did not expect her to have a sexuality at all, therefore her deviation from the asexual norm was not as significant as her deviation from the able-bodied norm (p.22).

Health and social care services: acknowledging individual sexuality expression

Health and social care services can greatly assist the lives of people with chronic illness or disability if in their care provision they can adopt '...a model of disability and sexuality which focuses on social processes such as expectations, imagery and barriers...' as opposed to one that '...dwells on individual impairments and biological differences' (Brown *et al.*, 2000, p.99).

Openness to individual sexuality expression or potential sexual need is essential if services are to be responsive and thus effective, as the following example from Brown *et al.* (2000, p.47) illustrates. A gay disabled man was living alone after the death of his partner. He was assessed for community care, and found 'all the disability stuff' difficult to deal with, in addition to feeling uncomfortable about having to justify his needs as a gay man. Later he found a new partner who was also disabled. When he was reassessed for community care he raised the issue of his unmet needs, and was offered residential care, with no thought being given to the implications. He was inclined to think that the authorities were making fun of him, and asked whether they had anywhere he could sleep with his partner, or who would assess his partner's needs if they spent the night together in residential care. Eventually he decided to remain in his own home, a decision which begs the question of the authorities' response to or consideration of his circumstances.

Sensitivity is also essential, as patients may not come straight to the point. They may fear looking stupid by using the 'wrong words', or in giving offence by being too explicit, or they have no way of conceptualising what is 'wrong'. A doctor can find himself or herself fumbling around in a slightly mad conversation in which nobody understands what is being said (Ramage, 1998).

Brown *et al.* (2000) recommend that openness and explicitness, however awkward, should be the goal so that the individual members of staff who support disabled people and who need assistance are not left unprotected and unsupported (p.99).

Building on self-esteem is also important. Body image, self-esteem and confidence play a fundamental role in the building and sustenance of relationships, particularly intimate relationships, and sexual performance depends on emotional as well as physical factors (Cooper & Guillebaud, 1999).

Seeing the positive opportunities

Some writers have found ways to convert challenges into positive opportunities. One woman wrote:

> 'I see my limitations only as parameters ... if you are a sexually active disabled person, and comfortable with the sexual side of your life, it is remarkable how dull and unimaginative non-disabled people's sex lives can appear. I am often left feeling surprised and smug when I hear my non-disabled friends bemoan the stale approaches of lovers, the tedium of flopping into the same sexual position, the lack of open and honest communication.'
>
> (Shakespeare *et al.*, 1996, p.203)

As the actor Christopher Reeve described in his autobiography (1998), many people with high-level or complete breakages of the spinal cord remain capable of satisfactory penile or clitoral erections in that the areas below the level of the lesion will respond to stimulation through reflexes, even if the person has no sensation in the area. Rayner (1999) also highlights that although some men with spinal cord injuries have to work unnaturally hard at getting an erection these often last much longer than before they were injured 'sometimes tiresomely so' (p.32). This is because the damage to the spinal cord prevents the brain's inhibiting impulses from reaching the cord below the site of the injury. For these men, orgasm can take on a greater significance. Bob Lenz, a sex and disabilities consultant, said that before he broke his neck, orgasm was solely ejaculation. Now he believes orgasm is more emotional than physical and that he is a better lover than before his accident (Bullard & Knight, 1991).

Addressing the wider issues

People with disabilities or chronic illness are disadvantaged if information and services are not made accessible to them in ways they can use. Mainstream organisations providing counselling and support about sexuality, relationships, sexual and reproductive health and the experience of abuse need to attend to issues of access, acceptability and presentation in order to ensure their services are as available to disabled people as they are to other groups. Services certainly need to be provided in accessible buildings, to have accessible publicity and to signal clearly that they are open to disabled people. People with impaired communication are often excluded from counselling. Counselling training should routinely include disability awareness, and disabled people should also be acknowledged in general sexual health material. Brown *et. al.* (2000) contend that services are patchy – 'there are islands of excellence within a sea of indifference'.

Conclusion

This chapter has explored a range of issues that impact on people with disabilities and chronic illness, but self-expression through intimacy has much less to do with sexual function than many people assume. Caring touch is what satisfies – giving and receiving it. Loving and being loved is ultimately a more powerful human exchange than raw sex and can be expressed in an infinite variety of ways. Peace (1996) suggests that while relationships are bound to change it is not always for the worse, with some people becoming closer despite the difficulties they both face.

Regardless of any disability, the human need for contact is innate. There is not a person alive who is not nurtured and healed by sincere loving contact. In this sense, a disability can be a gift. Once the ability to 'perform' in the stereotypical sense becomes limited, the focus can shift to gentler and often more intimate levels of sexuality. The pressure is off, and a couple can simply savour the truth of their loving feelings, as easily expressed through a kiss or caress as through genital sexual intercourse. Sex becomes more of an adventure, a chance to discover that there are many ways to touch, many parts of the body that are highly sensitive (Karp & Lamb, 1998).

Something special happens when we achieve an open, trusting and mutually satisfying relationship with another person. Intimate contact can be verbal; a relaxed intimate conversation can be very pleasurable. Most people are 'touch' starved and those with chronic illness and disabilities can benefit tremendously from the pleasures and joys of touching. Fondling and caressing sensitive areas of the body can be just as exciting and fulfilling as full intercourse.

People who have chronic illnesses and disabilities and those with whom they are intimate often have inaccurate or incomplete information about the impact of their illness or disability on sexual expression and they may know little about what options are available. Accurate information is vital in dispelling the myths and misconceptions surrounding sexuality. Disability and sexuality can no longer be described as one of our great taboos, particularly amongst healthcare professionals. Only when society can look beyond crutches and wheelchairs to realise that people who have disabilities are sexual beings, can accessibility become a reality.

As one disabled student in Brown *et al.*'s (2000, p. 64) study remarked: 'We'll know things have changed if they ever get round to putting condoms, tampons and mirrors in the disabled loos!'

References

Appleby, Y. (1994) Out in the margins. *Disability and Society*, **9**, 1, 19–32.

Bignall, T. & Butt, J. (1999) *Between Ambition and Achievement: Black young disabled people's views and experiences of independence and independent living.* Racial Equality Unit, London.

Bignall, T. & Butt, J. (2000) *Between ambition and achievement: Young black disabled people's views and experiences of independence and independent living.* Joseph Rowntree Foundation, York.

Borowicz, L.M., Goldsborough, M.A., Selnes, O.A. & McKhann, G.M. (1996) Neuro-psychological change after cardiac surgery. *Journal of Cardiothoracic Vascular Anesthesia*, **10**, 105–11.

Brown, H., Croft-White, C., Wilson, C. & Stein, J. (2000) *Taking the Initiative: Supporting the sexual rights of disabled people.* Open University and Joseph Rowntree Foundation, York.

Bullard, D.C. & Knight, S.E. (1991) *Sexuality and Physical Disability*. C V Mosby, St Louis.

Cohen, P. (1997) Tired of waiting: Chronic Fatigue Syndrome. *Nursing Times*, **93**, 6, 29–31.

Cooper, E. & Guillebaud, J. (1999) *Sexuality and Disability: A guide for everyday practice*. Radcliffe Medical Press, Oxford.

Corbin, J.M. & Strauss, A. (1988) *Unending Work and Care: Managing Chronic Illness at Home*. Jossey-Bass, San Francisco.

Fallowfield, L.J., Baum, M. & Maguire, P. (1986) Effect of breast conservation on psychological morbidity associated with the diagnosis and treatment of early breast cancer. *British Medical Journal*, **293**, 1331–4.

Glass, D.D. & Padrone, F.J. (1978) Sexual adjustment in the handicapped. *Journal of Rehabilitation*, **44**, 1, 43.

Hannah, M.T., Gritz, E.R., Wellisch, D.K., Fobair, P., Hoppe, R.T. & Bloom, J.R. (1992) Changes in marital and sexual functioning in long term survivors and their spouses: Testicular cancer versus Hodgkin's Disease. *Psycho-Oncology*, **1**, 89–103.

Hannah, W. & Rogovsky, B. (1991) Women with disabilities: two handicaps plus. *Disability, Handicap and Society*, **6**, 1, 49–63.

Karp, G. & Lamb, L. (1998) *Life on Wheels: A Guide for the Active Wheelchair User*. O'Reilly & Associates, Sebastopol, CA.

Keith, L. (1994) *'Mustn't Grumble': writings by disabled women*. Women's Press, London.

Kellett, J.M. (1990) Sexual expression in paraplegia. *British Medical Journal*, **301**, 1007–8.

Longmore, P. (1987) Screening stereotypes: images of disabled people in television and motion pictures. In: A. Gartner & T. Joe (eds) *Images of the Disabled: Disabling Images*. Praeger, London.

Maguire, P. (1989) Psychological aspects of surgical oncology. In: U. Veronese (ed.) *Surgical Oncology*. Springer Verlag, Berlin.

Morgan, M. (1994) Sexuality and disability. In: C. Webb (ed.) *Living Sexuality: Issues for Nursing and Health*. Scutari Press, Harrow, Middlesex.

Morris, J. (1991) *Pride against Prejudice: Transforming Attitudes to Disability*. Women's Press, London.

Morris, J. (1994) *Gender and disability*. In: J. Swain, V. Finkelstein, S. French & M. Oliver (eds) *Disabling Barriers – Enabling Environments*. Sage, London.

Morris, J. (1999) *Hurtling into a Void: Transition to adulthood for young people with complex health and support needs*. Joseph Rowntree Foundation, York.

Nissen, S.J. & Newman, W.P. (1992) Factors influencing reintegration to normal living after amputation. *Archives of Physical and Medical Rehabilitation*, **73**, 548–51.

Oliver, M. (1990) *The Politics of Disablement*. Macmillan, London.

Parker, G. (1993) *With this Body: Caring and Disability in Marriage*. Open University Press, Buckingham.

Parkes, C.M. (1991) *Bereavement: Studies of Grief in Adult Life.* Penguin Books, London.

Peace, G. (1996) More than meets the eye. *Nursing Times*, **92**, 33.

Pfeiffer, D. (1991) The influence of the socio-economic characteristics of disabled people on their employment status and income. *Disability, Handicap and Society*, **6**, 2, 103–15.

Potter, R.G. (1989) Chronic non-malignant pain. *Journal of the Royal College of General Practitioners*, **39**, 486–7.

Ramage, M. (1998) Clinical review of *ABC of Sexual Health. British Medical Journal*, **317**, 1509–12.

Rayner, T. (1999) Sex on wheels. *Nursing Times*, **95**, 36, 32–3.

Reeve, C. (1998) *Still Me.* Random House, London.

Rieve, J. (1989) Sexuality and the adult with acquired physical disability. *Nursing Clinics of North America*, **24**, 1, 265.

Roe, B. & May, C. (1999) Incontinence and sexuality: findings from a qualitative perspective. *Journal of Advanced Nursing*, **30**, 3, 573–9.

Royal Colleges of Physicians, Psychiatrists and General Practitioners (1996) *Chronic Fatigue Syndrome.* Royal College of Physicians, London.

Schag, C.A.C. (1994) Quality of life in adult survivors of lung, colon and prostate cancers. *Quality of Life Research*, **3**, 127–41.

Shakespeare, T., Gillespie-Sells, K. & Davies, D. (1996) *The Sexual Politics of Disability.* Cassell, London.

Sherman, B. (1998) *Sex, Intimacy and Aged Care.* Jessica Kingsley Publishers, London.

Strauss, A.L., Corbin, J., Fagerhaugh, S., Glasser, B.G., Maines, D., Suczek, B. & Wiener, C.L. (1984) *Chronic Illness and the Quality of Life* (second edition). C V Mosby, St Louis.

Turner, D. & Hughes, M. (1999) Common chronic problems and their management. In: H. Heath & I. Schofield (eds) *Healthy Ageing: Nursing Older People.* C V Mosby, London.

Webster, C. (1997) *Advice on sexual activity for people with chronic pain.* Pain Concern UK, Canterbury.

15.   *Sexuality Expression for People with Disfigurement*

Helen Roberts

The purpose of this chapter is to explore some of the issues related to sexuality expression for people with disfigurement. A number of different perspectives on human sexuality are explored in the earlier sections of this book and the intention here is not to revisit them but to highlight certain aspects. Particular consideration will be given to the influence of social and cultural norms, their relevance to an understanding of facial disfigurement and its impact on affected individuals. In addition some suggested strategies used to manage the consequences of disfigurement will be discussed.

Sexuality and conformity

Sexuality is an essential part of being human and encompasses a wide range of issues related to social and sexual wellbeing. Expression of sexuality is influenced by personal, social, political and cultural standards. Many of these are presented as norms in areas such as reproduction, sexual relationships and gender roles and legitimised through the popular media of art, literature and language (Bancroft, 1989). The representative power of social and sexual images and the pressure placed on individuals to conform to them is critical to our understanding of the expression of sexuality and disfigurement. The links between certain types of physical appearance, personality and social acceptance are very much in evidence in everyday situations. Whilst we might challenge sexual stereotypes as a serious representation of real people, their influence should not be underestimated. The pressure to attain the perfect body and thus project the right image can be so great that simply being seen to strive toward this ideal is enough to guarantee

226

both personal satisfaction and public approval (Tiefer, 1995; Grogan, 1999).

Through a detailed exploration of complex issues such as stereotyping, norms and conformity we become aware of the significant impact of physical difference and its effect on sexuality expression. An important part of this is the degree to which both individuals and society tolerate difference and the consequences for those perceived to be different or non-conforming (Grogan, 1999). Conformity, believes Tiefer (1995), is simply a code for being socially acceptable, the impetus for which stems from a strong desire to fit in. For example, efforts to appear normal can be seen in the way individuals and groups may adopt a certain dress code, behave in certain ways and even employ tactics aimed at hiding their natural differences in an effort to avoid exclusion and to appear socially and sexually attractive (Radley, 1993).

Sexual attractiveness, according to Bancroft (1989), is one of the most powerful assets human beings possess and mutual attraction between individuals relies on our ability to communicate feelings effectively in a range of social and intimate encounters. Within these encounters the usual communication patterns consist of a combination of recognised linguistic and non-verbal signs and constitute what Goffman (1969, p.16) refers to as expressions given and expressions given off. Whilst we predominantly use the spoken word to impart information, gain understanding of others and form relationships, it is estimated that approximately 90% of what we say is communicated through powerful non-verbal means such as facial movement, eye contact, touch and other forms of body language (Argyle, 1990). The ability to express ourselves clearly and favourably through verbal and non-verbal means is therefore a critical stage in the early formation of social relationships.

The cost of difference

Goffman (1963) believes that impressions are formed and assumptions made during the initial stages of communication. Many of these will be based on our immediate responses when confronted with certain types of physical appearance, language or behaviour. At this stage first impressions can become deeply entrenched and Goffman suggests that even when these are wildly inaccurate we continue to trust our initial judgement. We may believe our impressions are based on a valid assessment of the other person and be unaware of the influence of deeply held attitudes and beliefs learned from previous situations or relationships.

In many social situations the decisions we make about each other are based on what Goffman (1963, p.12) describes as a 'virtual' identity rather than an 'actual' reality. One particular aspect of this is *favourable* and *unfavourable* discrepancy (Herek, 1990). If discrepancy is favourable, i.e. the other person more or less meets our expectations and any disparity falls within the boundaries of 'normality', then we may overlook difference. Initial social contact is thus deemed successful. If, however, the level of unmet expectation and difference becomes too great and we are unwilling or unable to amend our view of the other person then communication can be impeded. It is at this point that the problem of unacceptable difference and even stigma, in its broadest sense, is likely to occur (Herek, 1990; Barker, 1999). Goffman describes stigma as '...an attribute that is deeply discrediting within a particular social interaction'; it arises when individuals' actual identity fails to correspond to their virtual identity (Goffman, 1963, p.3). Inherent in the attribution of stigma is the belief that the stigmatised person possesses either 'discrediting' or 'discreditable' attributes and because of these is excluded from full social participation (Goffman, 1963, p.14; Herek, 1990).

Goffman clearly outlines the consequences of stigma and explores in detail the assumptions upon which it is based. He considers the specific penalties applied to the individual which, whilst not always unkind, reflect the attitude and behaviour of those he calls the 'normals' and are based on a belief that the stigmatised person is in some way inhuman (Goffman, 1963, p.15). It is important to note here that Herek (1990) believes stigma in itself is not a problem but becomes one mainly in situations where the attributes of an individual are critical to others' expectations, comfort and perceived safety. So, for example, it could be suggested that severe facial disfigurement might not be a source of stigma in a Head and Neck Cancer Unit where a dramatic difference in appearance may be expected and be the norm. It can become a problem, however, when a disfigured person returns to his or her day-to-day environment and becomes an exception (Herek, 1990; Partridge, 1994). It is at this point that the full impact and reality of difference for the individual become apparent.

Stigma leads to the legitimisation of a range of discriminatory practices, including the use of specific descriptive terms, and tends to include the discrediting of any individual or group possessing similar attributes (Goffman, 1963; Katz, 1981). However, Goffman (1963) and others have shown that the attribution of stigma is neither consistent nor predictable. Both the negative and positive connotations of stigma serve as a useful social function; for example, stigma helps us to make sense of individual and collective difference by giving it a name. Katz (1981) believes that consequently, once named, difference can become familiar and perceived as safe and under our control. Overall, however, deviation from the norm still tends to be met with negative and sometimes hostile responses and can be seen, suggests Herek (1990), as evidence of individual and societal inability to tolerate difference.

So, in many social situations positive or negative inferences can be drawn from initial face to face contact and the potential for successful relationships rests on how we interpret, utilise and act on our immediate assumptions (Goffman, 1969). In a striking account of how first impressions can influence the development of meaningful contact the American psychotherapist Irvin Yalom in his 1989 work *Love's Executioner and Other Tales of Psychotherapy* explores an encounter with one of his clients. In a chapter entitled 'Fat lady' (Yalom, 1989, p.88), he describes in detail his personal feelings and reactions to an obese woman. His story provides testimony to the power of negative stereotypes, prejudice and stigma in a relationship. During the course of his professional contact with this particular client he is forced to examine a range of personal, social and cultural beliefs informing his perception of fat women. What follows is a story charting the exposure of his bias and the emergence of what Yalom sees is the 'real' woman, not the 'avalanche of flesh' he had initially perceived and been unable to get beyond in the professional relationship.

In Yalom's account of psychotherapy with this woman, important insight is gained into the extent to which we are influenced by assumptions and the potential consequences for all those involved in establishing social or intimate contact with another person. Many people who fail to fit in struggle to establish the kind of contact described by Yalom in their everyday encounters with others. Frequently this struggle is conducted in a climate of public prejudice and personal fear, particularly if, as with those who are facially disfigured, their difference is apparent and likely to be associated with negative stereotypes.

It is not surprising then to find that the majority of psychological problems disfigured people experience result from difficult social encounters (Robinson *et al.*, 1996). Negative stereotyping in such situations, suggest Newell and Marks (2000, p.177), often begins in childhood and can continue through into adulthood, with responses ranging from verbal abuse to expressions of pity being a common experience for the facially disfigured person. In a detailed account of the degree to which certain conditions in individuals or groups arouse intra-psychic conflict, Katz (1981) discusses the difficulty in attempting to analyse such individual and societal reactions to difference. As we know, positive feelings and behaviours may be extended to and reciprocated by people seen to be attractive, friendly and successful. This induces and reinforces a mutual sense of high self-esteem and personal satisfaction during social interactions. However, the experience for the person with facial disfigurement may be very different. Negative interpretations of their situation may contribute to a level of perceived threat experienced during the social encounter which can lead to feelings of fear and anxiety on both sides (Katz, 1981; Partridge, 1994). Naturally defensive behaviour aimed at containing this fear will follow. Barker (1999) highlights precisely this issue when detailing the nature of assumptions, beliefs and prejudice in relation to sexuality. Describing the 'great myth of reason' he illustrates how when people who do not conform to or validate our individual worldview confront us we often respond by vigorously defending our initial position and perceived threat to our security.

Barker (1999) goes on to explore how threats to established personal and social meaning often generate anxiety, which subsequently generates defensive behaviour. It is the enactment of this particular type of behaviour that ultimately reduces this anxiety and restores a sense of equilibrium and safety. An encounter between a disfigured and non-disfigured person may therefore result in defensive behaviour invoked by a range of emotions on both sides – these can encompass such feelings as admiration, pity, embarrassment, disgust, a sense of vulnerability and even the threat of dependence (Katz, 1981). To immediately express and act on these in a negative way may be deemed inappropriate and instead powerful behavioural norms are more likely to stimulate a mutually supportive, sometimes sympathetic, reaction perceived to be more appropriate to the situation (Goffman, 1963; Katz, 1981; Partridge, 1994). Equally, as Robinson *et al.* (1996) have pointed out, many non-disfigured people react positively to a person with facial disfigurement but the embarrassment and lack of experience in the social situation lead to communication difficulties and result in misinterpretation during interaction. As discussed later in this chapter, the relationship between the disfigured and non-disfigured person and the emotions 'difference' can evoke make it extremely difficult to identify true feelings, behave with clarity and create trust within the social encounter.

Seeing beyond the unusual

It is estimated that 400,000 adults in Britain suffer severe bodily or facial disfigurement either because of congenital deformity, trauma or disease (Robinson *et al.*, 1996). The challenges they face are significant, particularly if their impairment is permanent, immediately visible and interferes with verbal and non-verbal communication. Effective communication is determined by our ability to establish social contact, and is a determining factor in the development of satisfying friendships, intimacy and sexual relationships. Continuous exposure to negative, demeaning experiences in these circumstances can, suggests Partridge (1994), lead to feelings of extreme anxiety, self-consciousness, inadequacy and a sense of shame resulting in social isolation, loneliness and depression. If a person looks unusual, has facial restriction, cannot articulate words well or even eats differently then the process of communication, particularly in the public sphere can become awkward and embarrassing for all concerned (Partridge, 1994; Robinson *et al.*, 1996). Difficult feelings may be compounded by defensive and protective behaviour, which can lead to increasingly distressing and inept attempts at social contact. Social situations are reported to be the most problematic, not least because of the fear associated with initial face to face contact but also because of the uncertain outcome and potential implications for a successful encounter (Robinson *et al.*, 1996; Newell & Marks, 2000).

As suggested previously, difficulties in social encounters can lead to feelings of poor self-esteem and perception of worth and often mean an inability to communicate confidently. The impact of this may inhibit enjoyment in everyday social contact and prevent the development of personal relationships as a source of intimate and sexual fulfilment. It is important to note here that sexual fulfilment is not simply related to sexual activity, although the level of sexual responsiveness in another may affect our sense of worth and vice versa. It is sexual fulfilment in its broadest sense, as a vital part of self-expression that is of particular concern for all of us. As Webb (1994) explains, without the basic self-belief and confidence that stems from reciprocal sexuality expression it may be impossible to instigate the kind of initial contact which leads to a desired intimate relationship and the possibility of sexual fulfilment. Difficulties in communication, therefore, can lead to a cycle of poor self-awareness, decreased expectations and greater anxiety in relationships and result ultimately in denied need, defensive behaviour and further social exclusion (Goffman, 1963; Partridge, 1994; Webb, 1994).

231

The person with disfigurement will constantly confront these difficulties in a society where physical presentation is paramount. Interestingly, works by Partridge (1990, 1994) and Newell and Marks (2000) propose that neither the type of facial disfigurement nor the length of time people had lived with it relate significantly to the amount of distress experienced in the social encounter. What is important is the way in which disfigured people are able to develop the skills to identify and manage the fear, and reality, of others' reactions during social contact. Bury (1991) suggests that it is critical to understand the links between the nature of the difference, its visibility and the reality of managing it on a day-to-day basis. The individual's ability to cope with all of this will be based on his or her internal resources and previous experiences of rejection or loss. Some of the issues can be explored and understood within the context of what Partridge (1994, p.56) terms the 'SCARED syndrome' (see Fig. 15.1). This useful model outlines the feelings and behaviours experienced during social contact between facially disfigured and non-facially disfigured people.

You			They	
Feel	*Behave*		*Behave*	*Feel*
Self-conscious	Submissive	**S**	Staring	Sympathy
Conspicuous	Clumsy	**C**	Curiosity	Caution
Angry	Apathy	**A**	Awkwardness	Anguished
Resentful	Regressive	**R**	Rudeness	Reluctant
Empty	Excluded	**E**	Evasiveness	Embarrassed
Different	Defenceless	**D**	Distance	Dread

Fig. 15.1 'The Scared Syndrome' taken from Partridge (1994, p.56).

Managing difference

In an attempt to understand the experience of living with disfigurement it is perhaps useful to first consider the range of work detailing episodes of chronic illness, disability and life changes. For example, research described by Nettleton and Watson (1998) shows how unless we experience dysfunction, suffer pain or choose to change our physical appearance in any way we remain remarkably unaware of our own bodies. They describe the extent of this 'taken for grantedness' of the body in day-to-day life and explore the tremendous effort required to manage the process of adjustment, readjustment and adaptation involved in major physical, mental or life changes. This effort increases if underlying symptoms and their management are part of the consequences of a condition all of which, according to Bury (1991), reflect the reality of coping with difference.

Much can be learned about these experiences and the process of managing change, including the impact of being different for those with facial disfigurement. Understanding can also be gained by exploring work detailing the feelings and behaviours that emerge during the experience of loss and grief. Miller (1992) describes how in difficult life situations individuals strive to maintain a sense of normality by minimising or denying the day-to-day reality of their condition. Drawing on the work of Weiner (1975) she outlines such strategies as 'covering up, keeping up and pacing' which can often be employed as a way of hiding the signs and symptoms of increasing pain, disability and sense of loss (Miller, 1992, p.28). These actions enable the individual both to maintain their sense of normality and subsequently prevent curious questions from outsiders.

Similarly Herek (1990) has shown how stigmatised individuals maintain their self-esteem through strategies that not only help conceal their difference, but actively enable them to use it as a means of explaining negative social experiences. For example, disfigured people who experience rejection in a relationship may blame their physical appearance. By not blaming themselves but the way they look, the disfigured person may thus confront the painful reality of the situation without necessarily experiencing a lowering of self-esteem and confidence (Herek, 1990). This highlights the effort involved in projecting socially acceptable images and the mechanisms necessary for self-protection; it also implicitly reveals individual and collective attitudes toward those who either succeed or fail. As discussed earlier the many coping strategies aimed at projecting an image of acceptability and normality involve hiding, disguising or modifying difference, not only for the affected individual themselves but also for society as a whole (Miller, 1982; Herek, 1990; Radley, 1993). Radley suggests that failure to do this not only suggests an inability to 'bear the stigma properly' but can result in the individual being seen by society as less of a person (Radley, 1993, p.109). Critical to social acceptance and individual satisfaction, therefore, is the need to appear normal and make sense of personal experience in what might be an impossible situation (Radley, 1993). The evidence for this can be seen in constant attempts by individuals both to adapt to the demands of a healthy, or normal, society and to live with their difference without being dominated by it (Radley, 1994; Morse *et al.*, 1994).

Despite the fact that hiding and minimising may be successful strategies in disguising difference and maintaining a sense of 'normality', the cost to the individual is that he or she may continually anticipate and experience tension in the social situation. Partridge (1994) suggests that between 50 and 70% of people with disfigurement experience difficulties in communication, which can increase over time, especially if exposure to demeaning social encounters is prolonged. The degree of psychological disturbance experienced in these situations will vary and research involving people with burns shows 30 to 40% of them to be experiencing severe psychological problems two years after treatment (Robinson *et al.*, 1996). Evans (1997) believes that the visibility of the defect, how it happened, its temporary or permanent nature, the speed with which the change occurred and the prognosis or outcome all play a critical part in predicting successful social contact.

Price (1996) suggests that our level of satisfaction and self-esteem is linked to discrepancy between how we would like to look (body ideal), how we think we look (body image) and actual body function. Our sense of personal identity even extends, according to Helman (1984), beyond the bounds of our physical body to include other people, environment and invisible features such as personal space. Perceptions of these boundaries fluctuate with physical alterations. Thus, a discrepancy between any of these areas results in conflicting beliefs about our healthy, normal self and our damaged body (Helman, 1984). Failure to conceal, minimise the difference or overcome the resulting conflict may be interpreted as an inability to manage or be seen by others as a sign of weakness, failure and loss of control (Helman, 1984; Miller, 1992; Radley, 1994).

It is interesting, however, to note how perspectives on managing difference by concealment and hiding are increasingly being challenged. Suggesting that contemporary society has itself become more unpredictable, Kelly and Field (1998, p.15) believe that individual difference becomes 'just one more uncertainty' in a continually changing world. Seen within this context, managing difference becomes more about coping with it rather than trying to hide it. Indeed, they point to the many ways in which individuals and groups openly challenge society's negative attitudes to disability and actively celebrate their difference. For people with facial disfigurement, concealing strategies are unlikely to be a reasonable or realistic option; their difference is immediately visible and cannot be hidden. The emphasis then becomes one of finding alternative coping strategies and challenging social, cultural and political norms (Kelly & Field, 1998; Newell & Marks, 2000).

For the facially disfigured person it appears that much of the initial work in social situations relates to anticipating and managing personal feelings, gauging others' reactions and attempting to reduce discomfort (Partridge, 1990). Psychological difficulties in relation to communication appear to improve and be less evident in individuals who gain confidence in this way and are able to develop useful behavioural skills (Newell & Marks, 2000). It is highly likely, therefore, that professional support and skills training for people stigmatised by facial disfigurement can help ease the transition and difficulties experienced during the social encounter (Partridge, 1994; Robinson *et al.*, 1996; Newell & Marks, 2000). Evaluation of social interactions skills workshops shows how raising awareness and the development of specific coping strategies was felt to be beneficial in enabling the person with disfigurement to feel more confident in social situations (Partridge, 1994; Robinson *et al.*, 1996; Newell & Marks, 2000).

Offering support

Effective support of a person with facial disfigurement is only likely to happen in a climate of mutual and genuine acknowledgement of altered appearance. Hayter (1996) suggests that nurses are not immune to social and cultural influences, particularly in the area of sexuality. Exploring these and bringing other potentially difficult issues to the fore may encourage honest confrontation of the problems associated with disfigurement and ensure a realistic appraisal of the support needed.

In any professional relationship uncomfortable feelings and negative attitudes can be experienced, especially when addressing such intimate issues as physical appearance, sexuality and loss. It is often through physical touch, facial expression and voice tone that difficult feelings unintentionally leak out, are misinterpreted and cause discomfort (Hawkins & Shohet, 1989). Observing individual nuances within an interaction may reveal an individual's true experiences and feelings about a situation and the meaning drawn from it. It can also tell us a great deal about appropriate boundaries. Radley and Billing (1996) suggest that it is not simply what we say about our bodies but how we say it that sets the boundaries for verbal and non-verbal communication. Defining ourselves confidently in this way allows us to control how we project our attributes, protects us from admitting personal deficiencies and enables personal integrity (Herek, 1990). By openly and honestly discussing the issue of disfigurement within mutually agreed boundaries, both the nurse and patient can attempt to face the reality of difference at an agreed pace. The practicalities of this require a willingness to develop a range of behavioural and interpersonal skills and an ability to confront uncomfortable feelings and prejudice. Prejudice, believes Barker (1999), is learned, an act of will. It is not an instinctive response and to maintain prejudice requires us actively *not* to think and 'not to be open to the evidence or experiences that might determine a different outcome' (Barker, 1999, p.217). In his analysis of nurses' responses to the sexual orientation of patients, Hayter (1996) demonstrated that even where a level of awareness about individual prejudice existed, emotional distancing within the relationship still occurred and the effect on the patient was often one of feeling awkward, embarrassed and excluded. It is therefore perhaps incumbent on nurses and other healthcare professionals working with people with disfigurement to explore ways in which an individual's appearance might be a starting point, not a barrier, for exploring potential difficulties in social and sexual relationships (Partridge, 1990).

A significant contribution nurses and other healthcare professionals can make lies in recognising personal attitudes to disfigurement and understanding how these influence communication. Feelings ranging from compassion and pity to distaste, disgust and even hatred may emerge. Whilst the ambivalence of these feelings may be manageable for short periods of time, their meaning and purpose need to be understood and openly explored if intolerable anxiety is not to dominate communication (Menzies, 1970). It is precisely because of the difficulty experienced during some encounters that nurses may become conscious of previously hidden aspects of themselves. When this is not easily managed it adds to the level of discomfort and anxiety and may result in counterproductive behaviour. Developing the means of tolerating difficult feelings without the need to act immediately and recognising the meaning and purpose of defensive behaviour is crucial to effective communication (Brown & Pedder, 1991). Hawkins and Shohet (1989) believe that it is often because of our inability to avoid immediate impulsive action when witnessing another's pain and distress that inadequate or inappropriate attempts at solutions are made. As they clearly point out though, many people live daily with their distress and often have an ability to tolerate it far more than we who observe can. Recognising how we project feelings and experiences onto others, and resisting our propensity towards this, is just one of the first steps in developing the skills needed to 'stay with' the patient until they reach their own understanding (Hawkins & Shohet, 1989, pp.153–4). Being with another person in this way can often be extremely difficult, particularly if external factors such as workload, environment and lack of experience interfere.

It takes courage and insight to challenge, change and develop our usual way of doing things. Breaking patterns of unhelpful thinking and behaviour, and challenging external factors, can be difficult, especially if we are not prepared for and supported in the significant and sometimes unwelcome personal consequences. But, as Hawkins and Shohet (1989) point out, if we react to such challenges with unquestioning defensiveness we may miss the opportunity to develop a more genuine relationship with others. We also fail to recognise the potential for self-development and to explore aspects of ourselves, which may lead to a greater awareness of our attitudes, assumptions and behaviours when faced with similar situations, personally, professionally or socially, in the future.

It is important to remember that for individuals coping with disfigurement it is their individual, family and social life which is most affected (Noble, 1997). Within any of these contexts negative feelings often emerge leading to frustrated attempts at honest communication, anger, increasing isolation and reduced intimacy. Additionally, constant attempts to hide and minimise painful feelings can lead to an enormous sense of shame and perpetuate the cycle of fear and inadequacy in communication (Noble, 1997). Within the often limited confines of the nurse–patient relationship, developing specific skills aimed at exploring and changing behaviour may be an appropriate, and indeed safer, approach. The consequences of this, according to Bury (1991), will be in a range of responses. Some of these will be acceptable, others not. It is only with time and experience that the individual with disfigurement who is seen as different will learn how to live with his or her condition and others' responses to it. It is through the day-to-day living with their experience and appropriate support that individuals come to gain control and establish perspective on their own terms (Bury, 1991).

Conclusion

Coming to terms with disfigurement is an enormous personal challenge, and facial disfigurement in particular is likely to complicate social, intimate and sexual relationships. Rather than ignore this, it is beneficial in the longer term for all concerned to openly acknowledge such issues, however uncomfortable. Openness can be a sensitive way of actively using disfigurement to encourage initial contact and to explore difficult feelings. The challenge for all of us is to create a climate that enables the person with disfigurement to live in the real world. The skill for the professional lies in being able to do this using the right mixture of honesty versus fiction, balancing optimism with realism and acknowledging that to some extent no one has all the answers; nor can any one person make it better. The aim of professional help is not to create dependence but to willingly 'liberate the person from its receipt' (Partridge, 1990, p.78).

References

Argyle, M. (1990) *The Psychology of Interpersonal Behaviour*. Penguin, London.

Bancroft, J. (1989) *Human Sexuality and its Problems* (second edition). Churchill Livingstone, Edinburgh.

Barker, P.J. (1999) *The Philosophy and Practice of Psychiatric Nursing*. Churchill Livingstone, Edinburgh.

Brown, D. & Pedder, J. (1991) *Introduction to Psychotherapy*. Routledge, London.

Bury, M. (1991) The sociology of chronic illness: a review of research and prospects. *Sociology of Health and Illness*, **13**, 4, 451–68.

Evans, M. (1997) Altered body image in teenagers with cancer. *Journal of Cancer Nursing*, **1**, 4, 177–82.

Goffman, E. (1963) *Stigma: Notes on the Management of Spoiled Identity*. Prentice-Hall, Englewood Cliffs, NJ (1968 version Penguin, London).

Goffman, E. (1969) *The Presentation of Self in Everyday Life*. Penguin, London.

Grogan, S. (1999) *Body Image: Understanding Body Dissatisfaction in Men, Women and Children*. Routledge, London.

Hawkins, P. & Shohet, R. (1989) *Supervision in the Helping Professions*. Open University Press, Buckingham.

Hayter, M. (1996) Is non-judgemental care possible in the context of nurses' attitudes to patients' sexuality? *Journal of Advanced Nursing*, **24**, 662–6.

Helman, C.G. (1984) *Culture, Health and Illness* (third edition). Butterworth-Heinemann, Oxford.

Herek, G.M. (1990) Illness, stigma and aids In: P. Costa & G. Vandebos (eds) *Psychological Aspects of Serious Illness*. American Psychological Association, Washington.

Katz, I. (1981) *Stigma: A Social Psychological Perspective*. Lawrence Erlbaum Associates, New Jersey.

Kelly, M.P. & Field, D. (1998) Conceptualising chronic illness. In: D. Field & S. Taylor (eds) (1998) *Sociological Perspectives on Health, Illness and Health Care*. Blackwell Science, London.

Menzies, I.E.P. (1970) *The Functioning of Social Systems as a Defence against Anxiety: A report on a study of the nursing service of a general hospital.* Tavistock, London.

Miller, J.F. (1992) *Coping with Chronic Illness: Overcoming Powerlessness* (second edition). FA Davis Company, USA.

Morse, J., Bottorf, J. & Hutchinson, S. (1994) The phenomenology of comfort. *Journal of Advanced Nursing*, **20**, 189–95.

Nettleton, S. & Watson, J. (eds) (1998) *The Body in Everyday Life.* Routledge, London.

Newell, R. & Marks, I. (2000) Phobic nature of social difficulty in facially disfigured people. *British Journal of Psychiatry*, **176**, 177–81.

Noble, W. (1997) Social and material ecologies for hearing impairment. In: L. Yardley (ed.) *Material Discourses of Health and Illness.* Routledge, London.

Partridge, J. (1990) *Changing Faces: The Challenge of Facial Disfigurement.* Penguin, London.

Partridge, J. (1994) *Changing Faces*: two years on. *Nursing Standard*, **34**, 8, 54–8.

Price, B. (1996) Illness careers: the chronic illness experience. *Journal of Advanced Nursing*, **24**, 2, 275–9.

Radley, A. (ed.) (1993) *Worlds of Illness: Biographical and Cultural Perspectives on Health and Disease.* Routledge, London.

Radley, A. (1994) *Making Sense of Illness: The social psychology of health and disease.* Sage, London.

Radley, A. & Billing, M. (1996) Accounts of health and illness: dilemmas and representatives. *Sociology of Health and Illness*, **18**, 2, 220–40.

Robinson, E., Rumsey, N. & Partridge, J. (1996) An evaluation of the impact of social interaction skills training for facially disfigured people. *British Journal of Plastic Surgery*, **49**, 281–9.

Tiefer, I. (1995) *Sex is Not a Natural Act and Other Essays.* Westview, Oxford.

Van Ooijen, E. & Charnock, A. (1994) *Sexuality and Patient Care: A Guide for Nurses.* Chapman & Hall, London.

Webb, C. (1994) *Living Sexuality: Issues for Nursing and Health.* Scutari Press, London.

Weiner, C. (1975) The burden of rheumatoid arthritis: tolerating uncertainty. *Social Science of Medicine*, **9**, 97–104.

Yalom, I.D. (1989) *Love's Executioner and Other Tales of Psychotherapy.* Penguin Books, London.

Part 4
Current Approaches and Future Developments

16. *Facilitating Sexual Expression: Challenges for Contemporary Practice*

Isabel White

This chapter aims to explore ways of overcoming (or at least managing) the embarrassment and discomfort often experienced in discussing sexual issues with patients and their partners. In doing so it offers four levels of intervention in psychosexual care in order to challenge practitioners to consider their individual practice contribution(s), while practising within their perceived sphere of expertise.

The challenges that remain in addressing sexuality within everyday practice will be discussed within the context of both individual practice and the influence of managerial or organisational culture.

Psychosexual awareness: a contemporary nursing expectation?

As discussed throughout this book, sexuality is a powerful subject that can generate complex, and at times unanticipated, responses from individuals. Sexuality can be particularly difficult to address within nursing. Everyday nursing practice involves intimate contact with patients' bodies, emotions, relationships and lives in general. It brings together the professional and the personal in a delicate interface. Nurses are required to work within their professional code, but they are also wives/husbands, lovers, partners, heterosexual, homosexual, bisexual, in love, out of love, celibate, sexually active, sexually inactive; they also have a whole range of individual beliefs, values, difficulties, fulfilment and sexual desires (ENB, 1994). It is within this complex public, private and ultimately social context that nursing work takes place and that individual practitioners seek to define their professional contribution.

Factors influencing the integration of sexuality within nursing work

An increasing body of evidence seeks to explain why nurses and other healthcare professionals emphasise the relevance of sexuality to their everyday practice while at the same time experiencing discomfort and demonstrating a tendency towards avoidance when sexual issues are encountered in their work. While the literature presented here relates to research associated with nursing practice, there is evidence to suggest that medical colleagues also experience difficulty in discussing issues related to sexuality and for much the same reasons as nurses, principally lack of knowledge and embarrassment (Hawton, 1985; Weijts *et al.*, 1993).

A small Dutch study (Weijts *et al.*, 1993) used conversation analysis to reveal the 'expressive caution' used within gynaecological consultations where both patients (15 female patients) and doctors (5 male gynaecologists) marked potentially delicate or sensitive matters with a change in their use of language. This 'expressive caution' was characterised by delays in discussion of sexual issues, often until the consultation was about to conclude or patients would refrain from answering sensitive questions until prompted further to do so. Almost 50% of the patients who took part in the study revealed problems related to sexuality, having first presented other gynaecological complaints. Both doctors and patients avoided the use of 'delicate terms' related to sexuality and tended towards the use of vague language such as 'down there' when referring to the vagina, for example. Depersonalisation of language also took place, whereby '... ways of speaking which loosen the link between the person and her most private actions and bodily aspects', were adopted in order to distance the speaker from the embarrassment associated with discussion of such intimate information (Weijts *et al.*, 1993, p.308). It would be interesting to repeat such a study using a larger sample of medical staff, particularly to explore whether these communication conventions still operate where the doctor and patient are of the same gender.

Table 16.1 provides a summary of selected research literature from general nursing that explores some of the challenges to the integration of sexuality within nursing work. An increasing body of evidence related to sexuality also exists within midwifery and relevant subspecialties or disciplines of nursing such as learning disabilities, primary health care, care of older people, cancer care,

Table 16.1 Factors that appear to adversely affect the integration of sexuality within nursing practice.

Individual practitioner factors

Biographical factors: formal practice of religion (Payne, 1976; Lewis & Bor, 1994; White, 1994) family upbringing: traditional (negative) attitudes to sex (Hacker, 1984; White, 1994; Guthrie, 1999)

Restrictive views on sexuality e.g. contraception, masturbation (Hacker, 1984; Webb, 1988)

Heterosexist assumptions or restrictive views on homosexuality (Hacker, 1984; White, 1994; Guthrie, 1999)

Ageist stereotypes of 'asexual' older people (Webb, 1988; White, 1994)

Sexual stereotyping of nurses (Porter, 1992; White, 1994; Guthrie, 1999)

Fear or experience of sexual harassment (Hacker, 1984; White, 1994; Guthrie, 1999)

Embarrassment in discussion of sexual issues (Lawler, 1991; Wall-Haas, 1991; White, 1994; Guthrie, 1999; Meerabeau, 1999)

Discomfort in consideration of sex within the context of altered states of health, e.g. disability, mental illness, life-limiting illness (Hacker, 1984; White, 1994)

Not perceived by nurse as a priority of care for patient/focus of treatment (Kautz *et al.*, 1990; White, 1994; Guthrie, 1999)

Nurse perception of patient discomfort in considering sexuality issues (Hacker, 1984; Kautz *et al.*, 1990; White, 1994)

Lack of theoretical knowledge about sexual issues (Payne, 1976; Webb, 1988; Wall-Haas, 1991; Matocha & Waterhouse, 1993; Lewis & Bor, 1994; White, 1994)

Organisational/practice setting factors

Lack of privacy (Lewis & Bor, 1994; White, 1994; Guthrie, 1999)

Lack of time (Lewis & Bor, 1994; White, 1994; Guthrie, 1999)

---

coronary care, neuro-disability and rehabilitation. Some of this literature has already been discussed in Parts 2 and 3 of this book.

Early American research claimed a relationship between nurses' lack of theoretical knowledge about sexuality, conservative attitudes and a negative impact on the level of teaching and counselling related to sexual issues available to patients (Lief & Payne, 1975; Payne, 1976). However, an indirect replication study by Webb (1988) found only a weak correlation between greater sexual knowledge and more liberal attitudes towards sexual issues among nurses. Although Webb attributed this to problems related to validity of the measurement scales used, Lewis and Bor (1994) also failed to establish a significant correlation between knowledge, attitudes and subsequent practice. Another interesting finding of

Webb's (1988) study was that psychosocial aspects of sexuality were barely mentioned by nurses, with the main focus of information to patients related to physical effects of illness or treatment on immediate sexual function. In addition, much of this information was vague, inaccurate and left open to patient interpretation; for example rehabilitation advice to a 65 year old man after a cerebrovascular accident was to 'avoid stress'.

Most research studies related to sexuality in nursing from the 1970s to the early 1990s were surveys; many of them used previously validated questionnaires incorporating attitudinal scales or sexual knowledge measurement tools. This research approach, while assuring anonymity of response, may have lacked the sensitivity and flexibility to explore personal and professional attributes of practitioners in sufficient depth to uncover the full range of factors that can influence the integration of sexuality within contemporary practice. Interpretative studies became more prevalent in the 1990s, adopting data collection methods such as in-depth interviews, completion of clinical exemplars, participant observation or documentary analysis (care plans) in an attempt to gain greater understanding of the ways in which individual practitioners negotiate the complexity of sexuality issues encountered in their practice (Lawler, 1991; White, 1994; Guthrie, 1999; Meerabeau, 1999). As can be seen from the summary of findings in Tables 16.1 and 16.2, these latter studies do appear to elicit a larger range of elements from practitioners' affective domain as demonstrated through feelings of embarrassment, discomfort, expression of prejudicial views and the disclosure of sexual harassment.

Sears *et al.* (1988) remind us that it is the relationship between cognition (knowledge) and affect (feelings or emotions) that is predictive of behaviour (practice), rather than the influence of either component in isolation. This point is crucial if we are to identify strategies that will enhance nurses' provision of care related to sexuality. For a change in practice to occur it is likely that one would need to impact on the practitioner's affective domain, an element of our value system that is resistant to change because of its association with the emotions (Lewis & Bor, 1994). As will be discussed in greater detail later in the conclusion of this book, nurse education related to sexuality may have greater impact on actual practice if it promotes the exploration of values and beliefs held by nurses towards their role in sexual health care, alongside the less controversial provision of theoretical knowledge (Lewis & Bor, 1994).

It is interesting to note the apparent disparity between the proportion of available evidence related to factors that act as barriers to addressing sexuality within nursing and the relative paucity of evidence that helps us to consider how to improve the current situation. Table 16.2 offers a summary of some factors that appear to support the integration of sexuality within nursing practice extracted from the same literature reviewed in Table 16.1.

Table 16.2 Factors that appear to facilitate the integration of sexuality within nursing practice.

Individual practitioner factors

Belief that discussion of sexuality concerns falls within nursing role (Matocha & Waterhouse, 1993)

Feel comfortable and knowledgeable in discussing sexuality (Matocha & Waterhouse, 1993)

Education related to sexual history taking (Lewis & Bor, 1994)

Nurses of male gender (Lewis & Bor, 1994; White, 1994)

Organisational/practice setting factors

Sexuality perceived as relevant to practice setting e.g. primary health care, gynaecology (Kautz *et al.*, 1990; Matocha & Waterhouse, 1993)

Nurses experience repeated practice related to addressing sexual healthcare needs (White, 1994; Waterhouse, 1996)

Patient/client factors

Ability to discuss sexual concerns with others (Waterhouse & Metcalf, 1991)

Positive attitude towards discussion fo sexual issues with nurses (Waterhouse & Metcalf, 1991)

Client initiates discussion of sexual concerns (Matocha & Waterhouse, 1993)

Client and nurse are same gender (Waterhouse & Metcalf, 1991)

As can be seen from both Tables 16.1 and 16.2, the majority of studies appear to place the greatest emphasis on the knowledge, attitudes and practice of individual nurses as the principal determinants of psychosexual awareness and the actual provision of sexual health care. While the focus on individual practitioners is clearly important, an understanding of the impact of organisational and managerial culture, availability of health and social care resources and environmental constraints upon individual practice is also needed. There is also a paucity of research evidence related to patients' perspective on sexual healthcare needs and the efficacy of nursing provision.

Clearly there are a number of considerations in conducting

research related to sexuality in a patient population; some of these relate to the perceived relevance of sexuality to patients' principal healthcare needs. Other challenges are inherent to the conduct of all research in the field of sexuality, sexual health or human sexual behaviour. Detailed coverage of such issues, while relevant to nursing research in this arena, is beyond the scope of this book. However, readers are directed to Hawton (1985, pp.43–55) for a brief overview of methodological considerations in both general population and clinical surveys of sexual difficulties.

Developing psychosexual awareness: levels of nursing intervention

The potential role of the nurse in psychosexual care is both multi-faceted and diverse. The relative importance and precise mani-festation of specific aspects of the role will be determined, to a large extent, by the clinical context where nursing work takes place: for example a surgical unit, rehabilitation centre or family planning clinic (Matocha & Waterhouse, 1993). For nurses working with older people, McCracken (1988) recommends three aspects of practice which are particularly important in promoting the expression of sexuality and healthy sexual functioning:

- sexual education in respect of changes associated with normal ageing
- education relating to changes associated with chronic illness or treatment
- advocacy in dispelling the myths associated with age and sex.

With minor adjustment to reflect a specific client group, age group or clinical setting, these three areas of psychosexual practice are pertinent to a wide range of healthcare settings where nurses may encounter people with sexual health needs.

While all nurses should have a basic understanding of sexuality and sexual changes through the human lifespan, some nurse interventions require higher levels of knowledge and skills. For example, the assessment and treatment of erectile dysfunction associated with diabetes, or advice related to the management of dyspareunia resulting from pelvic surgery or radiotherapy would normally require referral to someone with specialist knowledge. There are a number of nurse specialists/practitioners now working at this level of psychosexual care.

Annon's P-LI-SS-IT model

Annon (1976), an American psychosexual therapist, devised a cognitive–behavioural programme to assist those experiencing sexual dysfunction. His work has since been adapted within nursing literature to represent the different levels of psychosexual care encountered increasingly within contemporary nursing practice. The strength of this model lies in its capacity to clearly identify the key contribution that can be made by all qualified nurses and healthcare practitioners in relation to the provision of psychosexual care, dependent upon their specific role and level of expertise. The model comprises four distinct yet interconnected levels of practice intervention:

> **P**ermission
> **L**imited **I**nformation
> **S**pecific **S**uggestions
> **I**ntensive **T**herapy

The Royal College of Nursing (2000) used the P-LI-SS-IT model within their guidance entitled: *Sexuality and Sexual Health in Nursing Practice.* This document includes a number of case studies that illustrate the diversity of nursing specialities where sexuality or sexual health issues may be encountered, together with discussion points for practice, policy and service development.

Permission

The challenge to all healthcare practitioners is to create a care context or environment that ensures sexuality is part of the overall healthcare agenda. As a direct consequence, people with sexual health concerns are then more likely to raise issues with those directly involved in their care or support. Creation of a climate of *Permission* can occur at three key levels:

- organisational level
- systems of care delivery
- that of the individual practitioner.

Organisational level

Care context or environment
Consideration of the physical resources available to practitioners and service users is relevant when there is a need to create areas for

confidential discussion of sensitive aspects of care such as sexuality. In acute care settings it is not uncommon for nurses or other healthcare workers to be faced with the dilemma of conducting such conversations in a draughty corridor, crowded outpatients department or behind 'soundproof' screens in an open ward. Privacy for such interactions is imperative if people with sexual health concerns are to feel comfortable in raising such issues for discussion. Practitioners may have to negotiate access to consultation rooms or other vacant facilities adjacent to ward areas in order to reduce the likelihood of interruptions and to maintain confidentiality. Environmental barriers to the creation of private space for sexual expression can be of particular importance in residential care settings such as care homes for older people or for those living with a disability, as the following example cited in Sherman (1999) shows.

> 'The Masons are in their 70s and, up to the time Mr Mason was admitted to the nursing home, they enjoyed a satisfactory sex life. Then he shared a room with three others and when Mrs Mason visited they walked together or sat beside his bed. Visitors were embarrassed when they came upon them in a passionate embrace. Moving Mr Mason into a single room gave them opportunities to be together undisturbed. Both were noticeably less stressed and his advances to female staff became rare.'
>
> (Sherman, 1999, p.99)

As can be seen from this example, a lack of sensitivity to the sexual health needs of residents can lead to behavioural outcomes that both diminish the dignity of the person and create a further dilemma for practitioners in managing what may then be defined as difficult sexual behaviour.

It is imperative that respect for the personal privacy of residents or patients in institutional settings is promoted through service user involvement in the design of facilities. Lack of privacy can also occur when an older person lives with their adult children or a person with a disability lives with their parents and siblings. It may be difficult when an older parent, or a daughter with a disability, has a sexual partner to visit to find a place to be alone without other family members around. Negotiating the Permission to discuss such issues within a person's home context normally requires detailed knowledge of the patient/client and family in question, together with a sensitive and non-confrontational approach.

Resource considerations within acute or primary care settings range from the availability of educational materials for nurse teaching about contraception to stocks of condoms in a GUM clinic. Young disabled people may be inadvertently denied choice in their sexual lives if information is not made accessible to them, for example materials for those with visual or hearing impairment. Brown *et al.* (2000) found that there was a lack of materials related to disability and sexuality within schools and that the resources available did not feature people with disability, thus reinforcing their social (and sexual) exclusion.

In-patient settings could create a more conducive environment for patients, partners and staff through the display of appropriate posters, patient information leaflets or useful contact lists of self-help groups and counselling facilities related to sexual issues.

The organisational culture of a service or clinical setting can reinforce the lived experience of invisibility, isolation or prejudice for individuals with sexual difficulties, particularly where they also identify themselves as gay, lesbian or bisexual. Nurses appear to adopt heterosexist assumptions when considering the sexuality of their patients (White, 1994) or express negative attitudes toward homosexual patients where their sexual orientation is known (Guthrie, 1999). Indeed Hayter (1996, p.663) argues '...that the advent of HIV has merely served to legitimise the expression of negative attitudes of nurses toward homosexual patients rather than create them'.

Heterosexist assumptions can result in the denial of access to information or to visiting rights for same-sex partners or lead to insensitive questioning during an assessment interview. A person may be asked their marital status when they are in an established same-sex relationship and may wish their partner to be identified as their next-of-kin. The Royal College of Nursing (RCN) (1998a) has published specific guidance on the legal status of 'next of kin' for lesbian and gay patients and for children with lesbian or gay parents. This and other related RCN guidance documents provide suggestions as to how both practitioners and services can become more sensitive and responsive to the needs of gay and lesbian patients. Practitioners are asked to challenge heterosexist assump-tions and homophobic views, to adopt inclusive language and to offer positive images of same-sex relationships within service information. Practitioners must also recognise the importance of confidentiality and privacy where disclosure of a couple's same-sex relationship may create difficult family dynamics during illness or at a time of crisis (RCN, 1994, 1998b).

As discussed in Chapter 4, many healthcare services perpetuate the 'invisibility' of same-sex relationships not only for service users but also for their own staff. It is important that organisations develop equal opportunity policies and care philosophies that both promote inclusiveness and are intolerant of prejudice or discrimination (RCN, 1998b). Through active awareness training and effective service development it should be possible to create a managerial and organisational culture that creates Permission for both staff and service users to be open about their sexual orientation where relevant and appropriate for individuals to do so.

Systems of care delivery

Systems of care delivery can also reduce privacy and opportunity for sexual expression. For example, if a woman with motor neurone disease finds the best time to have sex with her partner is in the morning, but this is also the time when the community nursing services visit to assist her with personal hygiene, how might flexibility of care provision accommodate such needs?

The documentation of care, particularly needs assessment, should be structured to include relevant information related to the sexual health of individuals, particularly where disability, illness or treatment may have an impact on sexuality or sexual expression. A young woman with learning disability may require sexual health education related both to the control of her fertility and to risk reduction in relation to safe sexual behaviours (Aylott, 1999a). A nurse working with such a client would also need to consider whether or not this woman was at risk of exploitation or abuse. Assessment documentation should clearly identify the need for social education about intimate and sexual relationships that incorporates strategies aimed at reducing the woman's vulnerability to abuse, while at the same time affording the woman the same right to opportunities to express her sexuality as others (Aylott, 1999b). Assessment documentation and core care plans in a unit where surgical interventions commonly cause temporary or permanent sexual dysfunction should include sections where appropriate to detail specific information related to an individual's sexual health, while still ensuring confidentiality. In this way the design of nursing documentation can enable the nurse to raise the topic of sexuality with patients as an integral aspect of their planned health care.

Care systems that promote continuity of care, such as primary nursing or key worker systems can both create and resolve problems related to sexuality. Such continuity promotes the development of rapport between nurse and patient and it is therefore more likely that the quality of the nurse–patient relationship will facilitate the discussion and management of sensitive care issues such as those related to sexuality. However, if the nurse in question feels unable to address such matters with an allocated patient then there is the risk that sexuality issues will be suppressed or ignored, resulting in needs being unmet. Indeed, as discussed in Chapter 4, such close nurse–patient relationships may also be a source of sexual harassment or abuse. Clearly, Permission must also extend to that of the nurse in addressing a knowledge or skill deficit, or aspects of sexuality in practice that are perceived as problematic, with their line manager or within professional supervision. It is important that those responsible for healthcare management systems and local healthcare policies can create the necessary balance between meeting the complex needs of individual service users and the inherent challenge in maintaining sensitive and responsive professional care and support in the domain of sexuality.

Individual practitioners

As discussed earlier in this chapter, there appear to be a number of barriers to the integration of psychosexual awareness in the practice repertoire of healthcare practitioners, one of the most pervasive and influential being the presence of negative attitudes. Such attitudes may be expressed towards sexual issues in general, to sexuality in relation to a particular care context or client group or towards the inclusion of sexual health issues within one's professional role. For example, stereotypical attitudes about homosexuality could lead a nurse to assume incorrectly that a woman who has had a hysterectomy may require less psychological support in relation to her loss of fertility if she is also a lesbian and is thus assumed to have given up her desire to have children because she has a same-sex partner. Another manifestation of negative or restrictive attitudes still occurs in some care homes where men and women are separated, even when they are married. There may be specific (usually public) places for mixed company to congregate and local rules about male residents going into women's rooms and vice versa. Such rules often go unchallenged but tend to indicate a less than liberal attitude to the sexual rights of residents when compared with the general population. Practitioners can implement aspects of good practice that maintain the autonomy and dignity of residents in creating Permission for people to express sexuality in ways that are both individually and collectively acceptable. Practice considerations may include:

- room doors being kept closed
- staff must knock and wait for permission to enter before doing so
- residents are free to remain in rooms and stay undisturbed
- facilities for privacy between couples/partners are provided
- giving consideration of the intrusion on privacy by staff members or residents of the opposite gender, particularly in mixed-sex care settings.

Many of these practice considerations are also relevant to the maintenance of patient dignity and autonomy within acute care, rehabilitation or palliative care settings. However, in acute care contexts practitioners can experience greater difficulty in striking a balance between the need for clinical observation, the rights of other patients, visitors or staff and the desire for privacy by individual patients and their partners.

Most importantly, individual practitioners can create Permission for the discussion of sexual issues by conveying to the patient that sexuality is an appropriate topic for discussion and in initiating such a conversation. A number of the studies reviewed in Table 16.1 found either a low level or complete absence of nurse-initiated discussions related to sexuality (Kautz *et al.*, 1990; Matocha & Waterhouse, 1993; Lewis & Bor, 1994; Guthrie, 1999). This is despite the fact that 92% of Waterhouse and Metcalf's (1991) sample of healthy volunteers thought that nurses should discuss sexual concerns with patients/clients. A significant number of research studies reviewed by Waterhouse (1996, p.416) provide evidence '... that most patients prefer to have discussion about sexuality initiated by health-care professionals, and that most nurses do not initiate these discussions.'

As discussed throughout this book, the reasons for this avoidance are multiple and at times complex (see Table 16.1). However, clearly there is a need for change if psychosexual awareness and care is to become an integral part of contemporary health care, as opposed to being viewed by nurses as a marginal activity solely for those working within reproductive and sexual health.

Limited Information

This level of intervention is characterised by the provision of non-specialist or limited information about sexuality or sexual health as related to the patient's principal reason for accessing health services. Within cancer care this may entail a nurse discussing the potential impact of specific chemotherapy agents on a woman's fertility and the need for use of contraceptive measures during cytotoxic treatment. For a practice nurse, Limited Information could relate to an explanation of the potential effect of a prescribed anti-hypertensive agent upon a man's erectile function. There are a substantial number of commonly prescribed medications that can have an adverse effect upon sexual function.

It is important for nurses to be aware of the sexual side-effects of drugs commonly prescribed within their speciality in order to provide appropriate patient education and to support the patient in seeking medication with a different side-effect profile where possible and desirable for that individual. The following list (Tomlinson, 1999) is not exhaustive, but classes of drugs that can cause sexual difficulties include:

Adrenergic receptor blockers (beta blockers)	Anti-spasmodics
	Anxiolytics (e.g. benzodiazepines)
Anti-cholinergics	Cytotoxic chemotherapy
Anti-convulsants	Diuretics
Anti-depressants	Endocrine agents
Anti-emetics (particularly metoclopramide)	Hypnotics
	Non-steroidal anti-inflammatory
Anti-hypertensives	drugs (particularly Naproxen)
Anti-psychotics	

In addition, one should also be aware of the adverse effects on sexual function of excessive alcohol intake, cigarette smoking and the misuse of non-prescription drugs such as heroin, cocaine or marijuana. However, it is often difficult to distinguish between the specific pharmacological effects of drugs and the impact of the often chaotic lifestyles of individuals who are addicted to such substances, including alcohol (Hawton, 1985).

As with the level of Permission, most nurses should be expected to intervene at this level of psychosexual practice. It is important, therefore, that the nurse is aware of the impact of physical or mental illness, medication and medical or surgical intervention upon an individual's sexual wellbeing. For example, why is it that some men with paraplegia can experience an erection while others cannot? It is beyond the scope of this book to describe the anatomy and physiology of the human sexual response, but it is essential that healthcare professionals have a sufficient understanding of this complex process before they attempt to offer guidance to patients. Readers may find the chapter in Marieb (1997) of some assistance on this subject.

With this knowledge, the nurse is in a position to support the patient through the provision of relevant health education, practical intervention and psychosexual support relevant to their immediate clinical need. Limited Information also includes being aware of the rationale for referral to specialist services available in the local area in order to facilitate access to psychosexual counselling or therapy where appropriate. Such services offer the continuing specialist support that is more difficult to provide within conventional clinical nursing roles and services. Specialist services may include clinics specialising in the management of erectile dysfunction, sexually acquired infections or counselling services for couples affected by infertility. Appendix 1 includes some useful addresses and contacts related both to psychosexual care and to the needs of specific client groups.

Clearly, in order to be able to function effectively at this level of care provision a nurse needs not only the theoretical knowledge to provide accurate and specific guidance, but to be able to discuss the sexual effects of a given condition or treatment without experiencing unmanageable embarrassment or discomfort. Irwin (2000, p.364) stresses that '...often patients will not expect the nurse to have the "answer" to their problems ... what a patient may require is the therapeutic space in which he or she can try to understand his or her feelings.'

The development of specific knowledge and skills in psychosexual awareness is discussed in more detail in Chapter 17.

Specific Suggestions

While the previous two levels of nursing intervention should be attainable by the majority of practitioners, the level of Specific Suggestions is more usually associated with advanced nursing practice such as that provided by clinical nurse specialists or nurse therapists. This level of practice requires not only a detailed knowledge of the impact of illness and disability upon sexual expression, but also specific knowledge about human sexual response and the nature of sexual expression together with its physical, psychological and inter-personal elements. In addition, such a practitioner must normally be able to demonstrate advanced communication skills and a personal and professional sensitivity and maturity that enables them to feel comfortable and relaxed when discussing sexual issues.

For example, a man with chronic obstructive pulmonary disease finds that his severe breathlessness affects many aspects of his everyday living, including making love to his partner. A specialist respiratory nurse working with this man and his partner could discuss the use of alternative sexual positions that may enable the couple to continue sexual expression with reduced respiratory effort. The nurse specialist who supports a woman recovering from a radical hysterectomy may advise her to try the female superior position in order to have greater control over the depth of vaginal penetration experienced during intercourse. In this way she may find her anxiety about resuming intercourse after her surgery decreases. A number of organisations now provide literature that illustrates the range of sexual positions that can be adopted to minimise the effects of muscle spasm, pain or limited joint mobility on a couple's sexual enjoyment.

Figure 16.1 provides some examples of alternative sexual positions that can be used when the effects of illness, treatment or disability require an adaptation to the couple's conventional sexual positions. While most of the patient education materials represent heterosexual couples, many of the positions are also appropriate for same-sex couples.

If a patient has an indwelling urinary catheter and wishes to have sexual intercourse, the catheter can either be removed and reinserted at a later point, spigotted and taped to the inside of the thigh for women, or placed within a condom for men. Insertion of a suprapubic catheter may ultimately be appropriate as a long-term management strategy for some individuals. For people living with chronic illness or chronic pain, sexual difficulties are commonly associated with fatigue and the resultant loss of sexual interest as much as the times when intercourse is too painful or mechanically impossible. Here the nurse can support the couple in exploring alternative methods of achieving sexual satisfaction such as intimate touching, massage, mutual masturbation and the use of sex aids, where acceptable. SPOD (the Association to Aid the Sexual and Personal Relationships of People with a Disability), BACUP (British Association of Cancer United Patients and their families and friends) and the Chest, Heart and Stroke Association (CHSA) are some examples of UK organisations who provide advice services and literature that specifically address the sexual expression of those living with illness and disability. These materials can be obtained for use by nurses in support of their direct work with individuals or couples, or can be offered where the nurse may only be able to provide an information exchange session. In this latter situation these materials can act as a point of contact for future discussion, referral or self-help.

See Appendix 1 for additional contact addresses and sources of counselling, support and information related to sexual difficulties.

As with all discussions related to sexual expression, it is impor-

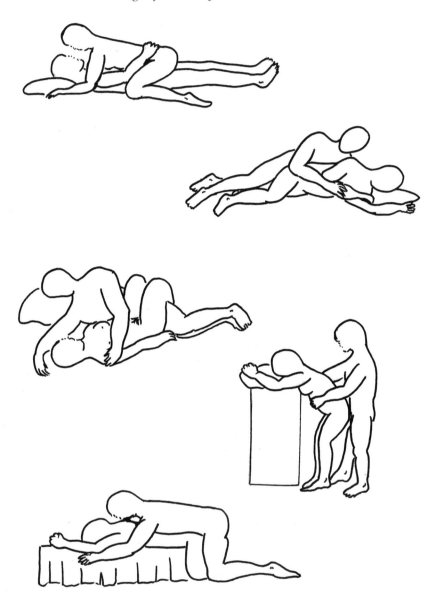

Fig. 16.1 Alternative sexual positions to accommodate the effects of illness, treatment or disability. Redrawn from materials produced courtesy of the Arthritis Research Campaign.

tant that the nurse is aware of what is likely to be acceptable and what may be considered offensive to an individual or couple. Such attitudes towards acceptability, as with sexual expression itself, is both varied and individual and is not necessarily determined by culture, religion, social class, gender, age or sexual experience of the individual or couple in question. For example, if the nurse is exploring alternative methods of sexual expression where vaginal penetration is no longer possible, would oral or anal sex be an acceptable alternative for the couple in question? Has the couple ever used sexual aids such as a vibrator to enhance pleasure in their lovemaking and would the use of such an aid be helpful now?

Clearly, one of the most important determinants not only of the success of the nurse–patient relationship in psychosexual care, but also of the resolution of many sexual difficulties by a couple, is sensitive and effective communication (Hawton, 1985).

Intensive Therapy

Generally speaking, Intensive Therapy is the province of those with additional specialist training in either psychosexual medicine or psychosexual (sex) therapy. In the UK, such specialist help can be provided within a variety of services within the NHS, voluntary and private sectors. Sources of help may be accessed through general practitioners, family planning clinics, genito-urinary clinics, clinical psychology, psychiatry departments, or specific sexual dysfunction clinics. An increasing number of nurses working in relevant clinical settings have undertaken advanced education and training in psychosexual medicine or therapy in order to meet the increasing service demand from patients and their partners. Some services require a referral from a medical practitioner whereas others may accept direct patient referrals.

The context of both the service and the 'therapist' does, to some extent, shape the precise nature and underlying theoretical perspective of the approach offered to individuals/couples. However, most contemporary practice in psychosexual therapy in the UK uses an adapted cognitive–behavioural approach such as that initially advocated by Masters and Johnson (1970) and Kaplan (1974). As a review of the range of approaches to be found in psychosexual medicine and therapy is beyond the scope of this book, readers are advised to consult texts such as Hawton (1985) or Bancroft (1989) for a comprehensive discussion of this topic.

Psychosexual work typically addresses the physical, psychological and interpersonal or relationship components of sexual difficulties, adopting an eclectic mix of behavioural, cognitive and psychodynamic approaches in working with individuals or, more commonly, couples. As outlined by Hawton (1985), Bancroft (1989), Irwin (2000) and others, psychosexual therapy programmes follow a detailed assessment of the couple together with a 'formulation' of their sexual difficulty and the possible cause(s). Treatment programmes are individualised to address not only the nature of the presenting sexual difficulty, but also the unique circumstances of the individual or couple in question. Most psychosexual treatment programmes consist of three principal components:

- education (or re-education) about 'normal' human sexual response and sexual myths
- homework (cognitive–behavioural) assignments designed to enable the couple to improve their communication and trust, to rebuild their sexual relationship and to uncover factors that may be contributing to the maintenance of their sexual difficulty
- counselling to support the couple in overcoming the 'blocks' or difficulties encountered during the homework assignments.

Table 16.3 provides a summary of the types of sexual difficulties commonly managed within either a psychosexual therapy or

Table 16.3 Common types of sexual difficulty encountered within psychosexual therapy.

Female	Male
Sexual desire disorders: impaired sexual interest/desire	Sexual desire disorders: impaired sexual interest/desire
Sexual arousal disorders: impaired sexual arousal (e.g. lack of vaginal lubrication)	Sexual arousal disorders: erectile dysfunction
Orgasmic disorders: anorgasmia	Ejaculatory disorders: premature ejaculation, retarded (delayed) ejaculation, retrograde ejaculation
Sexual pain disorders: dyspareunia, vaginismus	Sexual pain disorders: dyspareunia, ejaculatory pain
Sexual dysfunction due to a general medical condition, e.g. multiple sclerosis	Sexual dysfunction due to a general medical condition e.g. diabetes mellitus
Sexual aversion or phobias	Sexual aversion or phobias
Sexual dissatisfaction	Sexual dissatisfaction

medical context. Sexual difficulties can be classified as *primary* (always been present) or *secondary* (developed after a period of 'normal' functioning) and as *global* (occur in every situation) or *situational* (occur on some but not all occasions e.g. may occur during intercourse with a partner but not during masturbation).

Psychosexual therapy frequently uses physical devices, or pharmacological interventions, in conjunction with educational and psychotherapeutic strategies; working in partnership with individuals or couples towards resolution of their specific sexual difficulty. Such methods may include the appropriate use of sexual aids such as vibrators to enhance sexual arousal; vacuum constriction devices, transurethral or intra-cavernosal administration of prostaglandin E1 or oral sildenafil in the management of erectile dysfunction; or the use of vaginal trainers in the management of vaginismus. Surgical penile implants, vaginal reconstruction techniques, the use of male or female hormones and the repair of uterine prolapse, rectoceles, cystoceles or collagen injections to relieve urinary incontinence may all be appropriate measures employed in the restoration or improvement of sexual function. While outwith the scope of this book, psychosexual therapy may also be appropriate for individuals who have gender dysphoria such as transsexualism or for those who may be considered to have a paraphilia such as paedophilia or zoophilia.

Conclusion

This chapter has offered the practitioner a framework through which to conduct an analysis of their current scope of expertise in psychosexual care (P-LI-SS-IT model, Annon, 1976). Ideally, the focus of such an analysis should be the identification of appropriate practitioner intervention(s) together with an exploration of both individual and organisational development priorities that contribute to the provision of non-prejudicial, optimal psychosexual care.

If sexuality is to become a legitimate concern for mainstream health care, practitioners must develop '... a critical awareness [about] how nursing and other health professions can, both overtly and covertly, reinforce [the] oppression, inequality, disempowerment and expectations...' (Irwin, 1997, p.174) that surround sexuality, gender and power in modern society.

References

Annon, J. (1976) The P-LI-SS-IT model: a proposed conceptual scheme for behavioural treatment of sexual problems. *Journal of Sex Education Therapy*, **2**, 1–15.

Aylott, J. (1999a) Are we denying the sexuality of people with a learning disability? *British Journal of Nursing*, **8**, 7, 438–42.

Aylott, J. (1999b) Preventing the rape and sexual assault of people with a learning disability. *British Journal of Nursing*, **8**, 13, 871–6.

Bancroft, J. (1989) *Human Sexuality and its Problems* (second edition). Churchill Livingstone, Edinburgh.

Brown, H., Croft-White, C., Wilson, C. & Stein, J. (2000) *Taking the Initiative: supporting the sexual rights of disabled people.* The Joseph Rowntree Foundation/Pavilion Publishing, Brighton.

English National Board for Nursing, Midwifery and Health Visiting (1994) *Sexual Health Education and Training, Guidelines for Good Practice in the Teaching of Nurses, Midwives and Health Visitors.* ENB, London.

Guthrie, C. (1999) Nurses' perceptions of sexuality relating to patient care. *Journal of Clinical Nursing*, **8**, 313–21.

Hacker, S.S. (1984) Students' questions about sexuality: implications for nurse educators. *Nurse Educator*, Winter, 28–31.

Hawton, K. (1985) *Sex Therapy: A Practical Guide.* Oxford Medical Publications, Oxford.

Hayter, M. (1996) Is non-judgemental care possible in the context of nurses' attitudes to patients' sexuality? *Journal of Advanced Nursing*, **24**, 662–6.

Irwin, R. (1997) Sexual health promotion and nursing. *Journal of Advanced Nursing*, **25**, 170–77.

Irwin, R. (2000) Treatments for patients with sexual problems. *Professional Nurse*, **15**, 6, 360–64.

Kaplan, H.S. (1974) *The New Sex Therapy.* Brunner/Mazel, New York.

Kautz, D.D., Dickey, C.A. & Stevens, M.N. (1990) Using research to identify why nurses do not meet established sexuality nursing care standards. *Journal of Nursing Quality Assurance*, **4**, 3, 69–78.

Lawler, J. (1991) *Behind the Screens: Nursing, Somology and the Problem of the Body.* Churchill Livingstone, Edinburgh.

Lewis, S. & Bor, R. (1994) Nurses' knowledge of and attitudes towards sexuality and the relationship of these with nursing practice. *Journal of Advanced Nursing*, **20**, 2, 251–9.

Lief, H.I. & Payne, T. (1975) Sexuality–Knowledge and Attitudes. *American Journal of Nursing*, **75**, 11, 2026–9.

Marieb, E. (1997) *Human Anatomy and Physiology* (fourth edition). Addison-Wesley, San Francisco.

Masters, W.H. & Johnson, V.E. (1970) *Human Sexual Inadequacy.* Churchill Livingstone, London.

Matocha, L.K. & Waterhouse, J. (1993) Current nursing practice related to sexuality. *Research in Nursing and Health*, **16**, 371–8.

McCracken, A.L. (1988) Sexual practice by elders: the forgotten aspect of functional health. *Journal of Gerontological Nursing,* **14,** 13–17.

Meerabeau, L. (1999) The management of embarrassment and sexuality in health care. *Journal of Advanced Nursing,* **29,** 6, 1507–13.

Payne, T. (1976) Sexuality of nurses: Correlations of knowledge, attitudes and behaviour. *Nursing Research,* **25,** 4, 286–92.

Porter, S. (1992) Women in a women's job: the gendered experience of nurses. *Sociology of Health and Illness,* **14,** 4, 510–27.

Royal College of Nursing (1994) *The Nursing Care of Gay and Lesbian Patients: An RCN Statement.* Issues in Nursing and Health 26. RCN, London.

Royal College of Nursing (1998a) *Guidance for Nurses on 'Next-of-Kin' for Lesbian and Gay Patients and Children with Lesbian or Gay Parents: An RCN Statement.* Issues in Nursing and Health 47. RCN, London.

Royal College of Nursing (1998b) *Sexual Orientation and Mental Health: Guidance for Nurses.* Issues in Nursing and Health 48. RCN, London.

Royal College of Nursing (2000) *Sexuality and Sexual Health in Nursing Practice.* RCN, London.

Sears, D.O., Peplau, A., Freedman, J.L. & Taylor, S.E. (1988) *Social Psychology.* Prentice-Hall, Englewood Cliffs, NJ.

Sherman, B. (1999) *Sex, Intimacy and Aged Care.* Jessica Kingsley, London.

Tomlinson, J. (1999) Taking a sexual history. In: *The ABC of Sexual Health.* British Medical Journal (BMJ), London.

Wall-Haas, C.L. (1991) Nurses' attitudes toward sexuality in adolescent patients. *Pediatric Nursing,* **17,** 6, 549–55.

Waterhouse, J. (1996) Nursing practice related to sexuality: A review and recommendations. *Nursing Times Research,* **1,** 6, 412–18.

Waterhouse, J. & Metcalfe, M. (1991) Attitudes toward nurses discussing sexual concerns with patients. *Journal of Advanced Nursing,* **16,** 1048–54.

Webb, C. (1988) A study of nurses' knowledge and attitudes about sexuality in health care. *International Journal of Nursing Studies,* **25,** 3, 235–44.

Weijts, W., Houtkoop, H. & Mullen, P. (1993) Talking delicacy: speaking about sexuality during gynaecological consultations. *Sociology of Health and Illness,* **15,** 3, 295–314.

White, I. (1994) *Nurses' social construction of sexuality within a cancer care context: An exploratory case study.* Unpublished MSc thesis, City University, London.

17. *Addressing the Challenges: Agendas for Education, Research and Practice Development*

Isabel White and Hazel Heath

The previous chapters of this book have provided an analysis of both the societal and professional contexts that directly or indirectly influence the construction of human sexuality for individuals and thus for practitioners. These chapters also illustrate that in many ways contemporary society continues to view sexuality in such a way that its expression is frequently controlled, hidden, restricted and stigmatised, so it frequently remains problematic when considered within the context of healthcare provision.

On further scrutiny, the barriers to addressing sexuality within nursing practice generally equate with those prevalent within wider society. However, as Chapters 4 and 5 illustrate, the individual practitioner can experience considerable role tension as a result of the need to negotiate legitimacy of purpose within what may be considered both a public and private domain of human expression and experience. The discussion of thoughts, feelings and behaviours that may not even have been given voice between intimate partners is a challenging facet of nursing practice that requires sensitivity, confidence, a shared language, understanding and care intent or goal.

As discussed throughout this book, and more specifically in the research literature reviewed in Chapter 16, the principal challenges for practitioners, as they engage in the complementary processes of education and professional role development, are to:

- address inadequate knowledge about sexuality
- explore and modify conservative (usually negative) attitudes towards sexuality
- reduce 'discomfort' with sexuality
- clarify perceptions about the legitimacy and place of sexuality within nursing roles
- understand the relationship between practice context/speciality and integration of sexuality within nursing work.

While the above issues may appear to relate predominantly to the development of individual practitioners, it is essential to view education and practice development associated with sexuality in its social context.

Creating a responsive curriculum: developing knowledge and skills

In the field of sexual health promotion, Irwin (1997) rightly criticised client education strategies that perpetuated the mythology of individualism as a context for both policy and practice, thus ignoring the powerful social constraints that shape individual sexual health. Such a social context is also relevant to the provision of nurse education related to sexuality; no curriculum is designed or delivered in a neutral environment.

To this end, decisions taken about whether and where to place curriculum content regarding sexuality are both value-laden and political. Pryce (1991) and Irwin (1997) have both criticised the dominance of a biomedical paradigm for sexuality and sexual health practice, whereby sexuality is still taught predominantly in conjunction with obstetric, gynaecological or genito-urinary course content. While sexuality remains framed within the more 'respectable' context of reproduction and specific body systems, more diverse or less traditional definitions of sexuality are almost inevitably excluded. Thus traditional values and social norms about sexuality are perpetuated, reinforced and their restrictive impact obscured. For example, if sexuality is largely associated with reproduction within the curriculum, what message is conveyed to practitioners about the sexuality of an older person, an infertile woman or a gay man? Morrissey and Rivers (1998, p.489) would argue that

'...in the absence of a progressive educational philosophy that incorporates an affirmative approach to discussing homosexuality, stereotypic and stigmatic attitudes may well interfere both directly and indirectly with the care provided by health care professionals.'

The place of such content within any programme of learning must be given due consideration according to the overall aims, duration and scope (academic and professional) of the proposed programme. However, there is certainly opportunity for greater integration of sexuality within both the pre- and post-registration curriculum in order to challenge continued marginalisation of the subject in the eyes of both neophyte practitioners and specialists. Enhanced integration may be achieved through the adoption of a more progressive definition of sexuality and its association with curriculum subjects such as the evolution of gender role identity, development of social relationships, together with an improved profile within the context of mental and physical ill health or disability.

The curriculum in action: when practice makes (almost) perfect?

More importantly, the twenty-first century nursing curriculum needs to create space for discussion of the sexuality of 'self' and 'others', in all its diversities, not simply to increase the proportion of theoretical content on the subject. In this way, professional education regarding sexuality may begin to:

> '...facilitate the personal exploration of feelings, beliefs and attitudes to sexual identity [and] enable the professional carer to explore the relationship between personal experiences and beliefs and professional persona and behaviour.'
>
> (English National Board, 1994, p.6)

As early as 1988 Webb argued that nurses needed to develop appropriate communication skills in order to be effective in their roles as counsellor, health educator, patient advocate and referral agency with respect to patient problems associated with sexuality. She asserted that nurses needed self-awareness about their own sexuality and the effect of personal attitudes on professional practice and behaviour towards others. Webb also acknowledged the reality of being able to 'bracket' such beliefs as opposed to denial or the denouncement of personal values. In support of the views expressed by both Webb (1988) and Savage (1989) the authors of this book also reject the platitude presented in so much of the nursing literature about sexuality, namely that nurses must be comfortable with their own sexuality before being able to work with the sexuality of others. As this book and other writers have established, sexuality is not a static concept and we are constantly adapting to its changing nature as we evolve across the lifespan. In addition, as Chapter 4 clearly illustrates, feeling comfortable with one's sexuality remains a challenge when it is constantly being 'denigrated by stereotypes of nurses or by prevailing attitudes towards women, in particular, as sexual beings.' (Savage, 1989, p.28)

Grigg (1997) and Morrissey and Rivers (1998) concur with Webb's (1988) earlier work in placing emphasis on the greater adoption of experiential and interactive teaching and learning methodologies for topics such as sexuality. They advocate the adoption of a range of educational methods such as values clarification, case discussions, experiential workshops and seminars where personal and professional attitudes, beliefs and values can be explored in a safe and non-judgemental environment.

Waterhouse (1996) argued that nurses principally learn to become comfortable with sexuality in health care through repeated practice. She suggested that education programmes need to create the opportunity for realistic practice rehearsal opportunities such as simulated practice or the use of micro-teaching with video feedback. Alternatively, repeated supervised practice, particularly when supported by formal clinical supervision and reflection, can enhance practitioner confidence and self-awareness in this complex domain of care (Wells, 2000). The use of a specific seminar approach to role development in psychosexual care is explored later in this concluding chapter.

While the focus of this book has rightly been upon the development of practitioner knowledge and skills, Webb (1988) the ENB (1994) and Grigg (1997) have each alluded to the fact that lecturers also require support and development. Grigg (1997, p.62) is at pains to point out that 'The appropriate preparation of educators is fundamental to how the subject [of sexuality] is delivered'. In parallel with the learners that lecturers hope to inspire, the developmental needs of educationalists lie not only in the domain of theoretical knowledge about sexuality but also the acquisition of personal effectiveness in interpersonal skills teaching and the use of experiential learning methods. Subjects such as sexuality are often controversial, stimulate a range of powerful emotions, may be associated with mythology, misinformation and guilt and can provoke feelings of embarrassment, insecurity and discomfort. It is for this reason, Grigg (1997) argues, that educators need comprehensive knowledge, sensitivity and a complex array of skills in order to lead sessions and educational programmes related to sexuality successfully.

Professional role development: discovering psychosexual skills

At this stage of the book we hope not only that readers recognise the challenges inherent to psychosexual care, but also the rewards to be gained when both patient and practitioner have the courage to work with psychosexual difficulties, despite their feelings of discomfort or embarrassment. There are clearly many and varied reasons why individual practitioners do not always respond to the direct or indirect sexual health needs of people for whom we provide services or care. However, as discussed previously, if sexual health practice is to evolve beyond what is, for many, an unsatisfactory status quo, it is imperative we offer practitioners accessible and supportive strategies towards the discovery of psychosexual skills.

While the emphasis in much of the literature reviewed by this book relates to enhancing theoretical knowledge, there is also a need to challenge the '...Western education system [that] values knowledge at the expense of skills, and values cognitive skills rather than emotional skills' (Clifford, 2000, p.19). This concluding discussion provides a brief outline of one approach to skills development that is particularly pertinent to the enhancement of self-awareness, sensitivity and confidence in psychosexual care, that of Balint seminars (Balint, 1957; Balint & Norell, 1973). The Balint (1957) approach aims to promote learning through a greater understanding of the source of 'discomfort' present within patient–practitioner encounters. More specifically, Wells (2000, p.3) argues that:

> 'When a practitioner is aware of her own feelings she is often able to attune herself to her patient's feelings, and so begin the study of emotional experience and relationships that will form the basis of understanding patients' needs.'

Balint seminars usually comprise a group of 12–15 practitioners, with a seminar leader who acts as 'coach' to the group. The seminar process entails practitioners recounting the experience of an interaction with a patient and reliving some of the feelings associated with that encounter within a small group (Selby, 2000). The focus of the group's work is the study of relationships. The aim is to promote understanding of the feelings present in such an interaction through discussion of the shared experience held within the group. As a result of listening to such accounts, group members enhance not only their listening skills but also develop the ability to work with difficult emotional feelings that might previously have left them feeling overwhelmed. The role of the seminar leader is not to teach, but to promote and support a shared understanding and exploration of the feelings present within the interaction through 'reflection-on-action' (Schön, 1987).

Selby (2000, p.293) offers a summary of the nature and potential of reflective practice within a Balint seminar approach.

- Skilled practice that may be taken for granted is made visible, acknowledged and valued.
- As reflective practice is developed the seminar develops its own 'practice theory'.
- Recounting stories and the discussions that follow allow for clarification of the encounter.
- The exploration of the feelings and thoughts of patients/practitioners is revealed by unrehearsed stories.
- Support that is offered allows increased perceptions concerning the work.
- Knowing the how and why of an encounter leads to the practitioner being more flexible in approach (as opposed to seeking 'communication prescriptions').
- Knowledge sought by the practitioner is more likely to be relevant to practice.
- The leader's role is crucial to the focus of study and reflection in and on practice.

Such work supports the processes by which practitioners and teachers come to recognise the '...parallels between the teacher-learner relationship and the practitioner–patient relationship...' as sources of mutual understanding which enable practitioner, coach and patient '...to perceive their roles as part of a continuum rather than being separate and isolated from one another' (Wells, 2000, pp.313, 314).

This healthcare text (Wells, 2000) is to be commended not only as a detailed study of the complex interpersonal processes at work in psychosexual practice, but also as a resource that offers practitioner and teacher alike the opportunity to conduct their own 'action research' in the quest for greater psychosexual awareness.

Sexuality research and practice development: where next?

While this book has offered a substantial evidence base for practice, there remain considerable gaps, if not chasms, in what we know about human sexuality during states of health as well as in ill health.

While the needs of some patient groups may be relatively well represented, for example the sexual rehabilitation of those experiencing paraplegia or myocardial infarction, others remain underresearched and our professional awareness and response to their needs and desires remain inadequate at best. For example, what do we know of the need for intimacy among those who are dying or how to promote sexual wellbeing in a person disfigured by head and neck cancer? How do we respond to the sexual difficulties experienced as a result of mental illness or prevent self-harm in a young man with learning disability who masturbates excessively?

Not only has research to date generally not acknowledged the needs of the full range of healthcare client groups but some have been effectively excluded from studies. This has happened explicitly, as in the case of older people being excluded from participation in a recent national and supposedly comprehensive survey (Wellings *et al.*, 1994) because the upper age limit for the sample was 59. Exclusion has also happened more covertly, for example when people with disabilities have been unable to participate in research because the print on the questionnaire was too small to read, they were unable to hear an interviewer or physically unable to access a building to attend a focus group.

Developing a user-focused research agenda

The logical starting point is to develop research agendas that actively involve patients/clients/service users and focus on their priorities. User involvement is not without its challenges because of issues such as professional boundaries; power and control; knowledge, skills, expertise among both users and professionals in collaborative working, and attitudes among professionals towards service users as partners (Owen & Harding, 2000). Increasingly, however, service users are wanting to take a more active role in influencing the health care they receive and, rather than being passive recipients of care, working as partners with health professionals. In addition, there is currently a strong political momentum for involving service users and their supporters or advocates in order to ensure the most appropriate and best quality services (The NHS Plan, DoH, 2000).

Challenges in user involvement can be overcome. For example, AgeNet and the Royal College of Nursing developed a user-focused research agenda for nursing with older people (1999), and the Beth Johnson Foundation supported older people in developing their health promotion booklet *Healthy Sex Forever* (Beth Johnson Foundation, 1996).

It is important that methodologies are constructed so that studies facilitate the inclusion of service users, in all their diversity, for example people in a range of settings, not just hospitals; people with mental health needs or learning disabilities (not only through third parties and advocates but through newly developing techniques of narratives, informal conversations and group discussions); people from all backgrounds and ethnic groups (Thornton, 2000; Vincent *et al.*, 2000). Carter and Beresford (2000) identified two issues that are a key to full involvement of users:

- access, not only physical access, but an understanding of structures, arrangements and ways of working
- support to help people develop confidence, assertiveness and skills to participate fully, effectively and on their own terms.

Priority areas for research and practice development

The chapters in this book have highlighted a wide range of issues and questions related to sexuality in both clinical practice and education. These could help to inform and prioritise research agendas. There remain, however, many issues of both practice and education in which further research is necessary.

Practice issues requiring further research include:

- Enhancing our understanding of patient/client/user perspectives and experiences, particularly for people outside the conventional research groups of patients in gynaecology and genitourinary practice.
- Studying the effect of social and organisational culture change on the promotion of improved psychosexual practice. Research to date has emphasised individual practitioner issues and responsibilities.
- Evaluating specific strategies or interventions that enhance practitioner functioning in sensitive aspects of practice. Research has tended to focus on barriers to integrating sexuality in practice.
- Researching nurse–patient communication on intimate or sensitive subjects such as sexuality and identifying the determinants of enhanced 'comfort' in such conversations.
- Investigating the impact of gender on addressing sexual issues in practice. The needs of men are generally ill-understood, particularly the emotional impact of sexual difficulties.
- Designing studies that address the affective domain of practice (feelings, emotions, attitudes) and its relationship with psychosexual practice behaviour.

- When nurses do offer psychosexual care, how do we evaluate which interventions are deemed to be most effective and how should we measure such effectiveness? Can this be done realistically? As Irwin (1997) laments, even in the wake of AIDS there has been inadequate evaluative research regarding the effectiveness of nursing interventions designed to promote sexual health.

Education issues requiring further research include:

- Considering evaluation research into education and training techniques (e.g. seminar training, experiential learning) that stimulate exploration of feelings and emotions. The dominant focus in research to date has been on the attainment of theoretical knowledge and there is clearly a poor correlation between sexuality knowledge and the incorporation of psychosexual practice in everyday nursing work.
- Further research is also needed to evaluate the types of formal and informal learning experiences that lead to desired professional behaviours related to psychosexual practice (Gamel *et al.*, 1993; Waterhouse, 1996). Such research needs to determine the most effective teaching strategies or learner experiences that contribute to increased comfort for practitioners, thus increasing the likelihood that nurses will initiate discussions about sexuality with patients. (Webb, 1988; Gamel *et al.*, 1993).

Conclusion

Perhaps it is the very nature of the concept, as we both individually and collectively experience it, that makes the detailed and sensitive study of sexuality such a challenge for contemporary practice, education and research in nursing and health care. While this book has offered a considerable evidence base regarding this fascinating topic, there is still much to be learned. The primary aim of nurses, and other health and social care workers, should be the creation of an environment that is tolerant of and conducive to the continuity of sexual expression and intimacy for those for whom sexuality constitutes an important aspect of their lives. However, engaging with issues of sexuality, both our own and those of others, will continue to be challenging. Sexuality remains a source of deep and powerful emotions, from fear and embarrassment to infinite happiness and fulfilment. By facing the challenges and engaging with the issues at least we are attempting to enhance our understanding and, through this, to offer help which is more sensitive, appropriate to individuals, and ultimately effective. In the realities of contemporary society, sexuality will continue to be an ever-present factor in our lives, whether we choose to actively associate with it or not (Hawkes, 1996).

References

Balint, M. (1957) The doctor, his patient and the illness. Cited in *Caring for Sexuality in Health and Illness* (2000) (ed. D. Wells). Churchill Livingstone, London.

Balint, E. & Norell, J.S. (eds) (1973) *Six Minutes for the Patient*. Cited in *Caring for Sexuality in Health and Illness* (2000) (ed. D. Wells). Churchill Livingstone, London.

Beth Johnson Foundation (1996) *Healthy Sex Forever*. Beth Johnson Foundation, Stoke-on-Trent.

Carter, T. & Beresford, P. (2000) *Age and Change: Models of Involvement for Older People*. Joseph Rowntree Foundation, York.

Clifford, D. (2000) Professional awareness in psychosexual care. In: *Caring for Sexuality in Health and Illness* (ed. D. Wells). Churchill Livingstone, London.

Department of Health (2000) *The NHS Plan: A Plan for Investment: A plan for reform*. DoH, London.

ENB (1994) *Sexual health education and training, guidelines for good practice in the teaching of nurses, midwives and health visitors*. English National Board for Nursing, Midwifery and Health Visiting, London.

Gamel, C., Davis, B.D. & Hengeveld, M. (1993) Nurses' provision of teaching and counselling on sexuality: a review of the literature. *Journal of Advanced Nursing*, **18**, 8, 1219–27.

Grigg, E. (1997) Guidelines for teaching about sexuality. *Nurse Education Today*, **17**, 62–6.

Hawkes, G. (1996) *A Sociology of Sex and Sexuality*. Open University Press, Milton Keynes.

Irwin, R. (1997) Sexual health promotion and nursing. *Journal of Advanced Nursing*, **25**, 170–77.

Morrissey, M. & Rivers, I. (1998) Applying the Mims-Swenson sexual health model to nurse education: offering an alternative focus on sexuality and health care. *Nurse Education Today*, **18**, 488–95.

Owen, T. & Harding, T (2000) *Involvement of Older People in Primary Care Groups*. Help the Aged, London.

Pryce, A. (1991) Sexuality and the patient. *Nursing*, **4**, 44, 15–16.

Savage, J. (1989) Sexuality: an uninvited guest. *Nursing Times*, **85**, 5, 25–8.

Schön, D. (1987) *Educating the Reflective Practitioner*. Jossey-Bass, London.

Selby, J. (2000) Reflective practices and action research in Balint seminars. In: *Caring for Sexuality in Health and Illness* (ed. D. Wells). Churchill Livingstone, London.

Thornton, P. (2000) *Older people speaking out: developing opportunities for influence*. Joseph Rowntree Foundation, York.

Vincent, C., Riddell, J. & Shmueli, A. (2000) *Sexuality and the Older Woman: A Literature Review*. Pennell Initiative for Women's Health. Tavistock Marital Studies Institute, London.

Waterhouse, J. (1996) Nursing practice related to sexuality: A review and recommendations. *Nursing Times Research*, **1**, 6, 412–18.

Webb, C. (1988) A study of nurses' knowledge and attitudes about sexuality in health care. *International Journal of Nursing Studies*, **25**, 3, 235–44.

Wellings, K., Field, J., Johnson, A.M. & Wadsworth, J. (1994) *Sexual Behaviour in Britain. The national survey of sexual attitudes and lifestyles*. Penguin Books, Harmondsworth.

Wells, D. (2000) (ed.) *Caring for Sexuality in Health and Illness*. Churchill Livingstone, London.

Appendix 1. *Useful Addresses and Contacts*

Ann Craft Trust (formerly the National Association for the Protection from Abuse of Adults and Children with Learning Disabilities, NAPSAC)
Centre for Social Work
University of Nottingham
University Park
Nottingham
NG7 2RD
Tel: 0115 951 5400

Arthritis Care
18 Stephenson Way
London
NW1 2HD
Tel: 020 7380 6500
08088 004050 (freephone)

Association for the Sexual and Personal Relationships of People with a Disability (SPOD)
286 Camden Road
London
N7 0BJ
Tel: 020 7607 8851

Association of Psychosexual Nursing
PO Box 2762
London
W1A 5HQ

British Association for Counselling and Psychotherapy (BAC)
1 Regent Place
Rugby
Warks
Tel: 0870 443 5252
Information Line 01788 578328

British Association for Sexual and Relationship Therapy (BASRT)
PO Box 13686
London
SW20 9ZH

British Association for the Study and Prevention of Child Abuse and Neglect (BASPCAN)
10 Priory Street
York
YO1 1EZ
Tel: 01904 613605

British Menopause Society
36 West Street
Marlow
Bucks
SL2 2NB
Tel: 01628 890199

Brook Advisory Centres
Education and Publications Unit
165 Gray's Inn Road
London
WC1X 8UD
Tel: 020 7833 8488

CONSENT (Sexuality training for people with learning disability)
Woodside Road
Abbots Langley
Herts
WD5 0HT
Tel: 01923 670793

The Contraceptive Service
Tel: 020 7837 4044

DISCERN (Counselling & Therapy Service)
Suite 6
Clarendon Chambers
Clarendon Street
Nottingham
NG1 5LN
Tel: 0115 947 4147

FPA (formerly the Family Planning Association)
2–12 Pentonville Road
London
N1 9FP
Tel: 020 7837 5432/020 7923 5232

The Gender Trust (a registered UK charity that supports people who are transsexual, gender dysphoric or transgenderist)
PO Box 3192
Brighton
BN1 3WR
Tel: 07000 790437

The Impotence Association Helpline
Tel: 020 8767 7791

Institute of Psychosexual Medicine
11 Chandos Street
London
W1M 1DE
Tel: 020 7580 0631

London Lesbian & Gay Switchboard
PO Box 7324
London
N1 9QS
Tel: 020 7837 7324

Marie Stopes International
108 Whitfield Street
London
W1P 0BE
Tel: 020 7388 0662

Mencap National Centre
123 Golden Lane
London
EC1Y 0RT
Tel: 020 7454 0454

Men's Health Helpline
Tel: 0208 995 4448

MIND
Granta House
Broadway
London
E15 4BQ
Tel: 020 8519 2122

National AIDS Helpline
Tel: 0800 567123
Bengali, Gujerati, Hindi, Punjabi, Urdu 0800 28222445
Cantonese 0800 2822446
Arabic 0800 2822447

The National Back Pain Association
The Old Office Block
Elmtree Road
Teddington
Middlesex
TW11 8ST

RELATE (National Marriage Guidance)
Herbert Gray College
Little Church Street
Rugby
Warks
CV21 5AP
Tel: 01788 573241

SexWare (sexual aids mail order service for people living with disability)
PO Box 1078
East Oxford DO
Oxon
OX4 5JE

Sexwise
Chief Publicity Officer
DOH
Room 579D
Skipton House
80 London Road
London
SE1 6LH
Free Helpline for Teenagers: Tel: 0800 282930

The Stroke Association
CHSA House
Whitecross Street
London
EC1Y 8JJ
Tel: 020 7490 7999

Terence Higgins Trust
52 Gray's Inn Road
London
WC1X 8JU
Tel: 020 7242 1010 (Helpline)
    020 7831 0330 (Admin)

Turner Syndrome Society
2 Mayfield Avenue
London
W4 1PW
Tel: 020 8995 0257/0994

Women's Health Concern
PO Box 1629
London
W8 6AU
Tel: 020 8780 3007 (counselling line)

Index